This book is intended as a collection of herbal recipes and as an aid in understanding the various theories and practices underlying their preparation. This book does not represent an endorsement or guarantee as to the efficacy of any recipe or its preparation, nor is the book intended in any way as a replacement for medical consultation and treatment where such services may be required.

For
Mertianna, Eric,
Jennifer and Benjamin

We would like to thank all of the people who have helped during the process of compiling this book. Many gave valuable advice, encouragement, and even advance financial support to an unpublished author and a tireless healer. If we have inadvertantly left anyone out, we trust that this acknowledgement will serve as our thanks. A special thanks goes to Jim Lawton, Henry Poirot, Batyah Janowski, Adelaide Teague, Sylvia Sandifer, Michael Meyer, Nancy Kleban, Steve Brown, Barbara Apffel-Pierce and Jerry Apffel-Pierce.

We would also like to thank Mrs. Morrie Blake, herbalist and cosmetologist, for her help since the first printing.

Five years ago, I met Mildred jackson and began to work and study with her. i had dabbled in herbal medicine before, but had never encountered anyone who possessed so vast an understanding of the healing process. I tried to convince her to write a book to record and share her knowledge, but she would only wisely assure me that someday it would be done. Since that time I have attended hundreds of classes and recorded remedies from thousands of sources. Mildred and I have experimented and carefully selected the remedies which appear here. In almost all cases, these formulas have been used by one of us or by close friends, and are safe and effective when used properly.

During this time, I have gained a tremendous respect for the resiliency of the body as it undergoes the constant struggle to maintain it's many balances. This book is an attempt to share knowledge and awaken that respect in others who may have lost contact with the natural elements.

Terri Teague

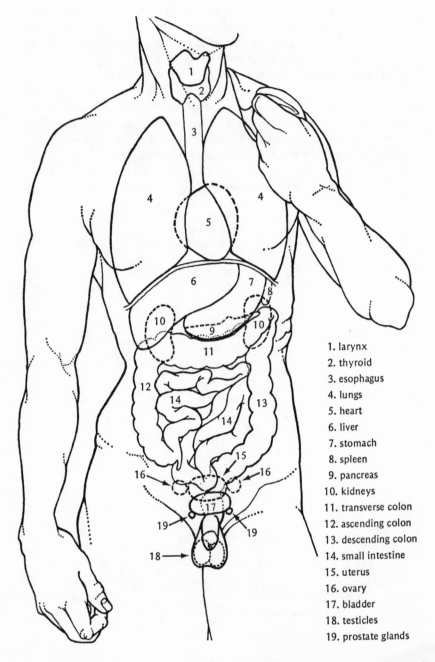

1. larynx
2. thyroid
3. esophagus
4. lungs
5. heart
6. liver
7. stomach
8. spleen
9. pancreas
10. kidneys
11. transverse colon
12. ascending colon
13. descending colon
14. small intestine
15. uterus
16. ovary
17. bladder
18. testicles
19. prostate glands

INTERNAL ORGANS

THE HANDBOOK OF ALTERNATIVES TO CHEMICAL MEDICINE

MILDRED JACKSON, N. D./TERRI TEAGUE

TABLE OF CONTENTS

introduction. vii

frontispiece viii

Chapter 1   Guidelines to Health 5

Chapter 2   Guides to Preparation. 11

Chapter 3   Remedies. 15

                        Arthritis, Bursitis and Rheumatism. 16

                        Backaches 19

                        Brain 20

                        Cancer 28

                        Chronic Diseases 31

                        Coughs and Colds. 35

                        Digestive System 46

                        Ears. 57

                        Eyes 59

                        Feet and Legs 66

                        Female 69

                        Glandular System. 77

                        Headaches 80

                        Heart and Circulatory System. 81

                        High and Low Blood Pressure 87

                        Insects 90

                        Kidney and Bladder. 93

                        Liver and Spleen 97

                        Male 102

                        Skin. 104

                        Teeth and Gums. 119

                        Weight 122

                        Worms 125

Chapter 4   Emergency Procedures 128

Chapter 5   Fasting 133

Chapter 6   Plants and Pets 137

Appendices

                       143

                        Elements and Minerals 144

                        Vitamins. 148

                        Hand Chart 152

                        Herbal Sources 153

References 155

Index 161

About the Authors 179

CHAPTER 1

GUIDELINES TO HEALTH

GUIDELINES
TO HEALTH

A properly functioning body is no accident. It is the result of consumption of the proper foods, adequate exercise, and regulation of your environment. All organs of the body are interrelated, and a malfunction in one will create disturbance in all of the others. You must become familiar with your body and its needs. Each one mends at a different rate as we are each physically and chemically unique, and requirements for nourishment, exercise, and environment vary from individual to individual.

It is important to remember that the harmony of health, and not the disharmony of disease, is the "normal" state of the body. Achievement of this "normal" state is made difficult by our fast paced society, the primary by-products of which are tension, confusion and pressure. Yet in the face of these distractions, each person bears the responsibility for his or her health and that of his or her children and charges. It is comforting to know that there is a simple and inexpensive alternative to high blood pressure and high medical and pharmaceutical bills.

THINKING

Worry and fear are major causes of disease, and psychosomatic illnesses are as painful and uncomfortable as organic ones. In fact, anxiety over disease can not only make you think you are ill, but can actually make you ill! Many parents inadvertantly encourage illness in their children by over-reacting. If you tell your child that he or she is going to catch a cold, you are encouraging disease rather than health. On the other hand, parents can promote health and facilitate healing by encouraging their children to be well.

Many of us worry about major misfortune and, in doing so, create stresses which deplete our reserves of vitamins and minerals. If your body is allowed to function properly you will not only be less likely to think about being ill, but your natural resistance will protect you from sickness. Alfalfa or red clover, taken daily in tablet or tea form, will restore a high level of resistance. Colds, flu, and even children's diseases such as mumps and measles can be avoided if the body resistance is kept high.

Anger, dissatisfaction and negativity inhibit the body's ability to function naturally, and create an atmosphere within the body conducive to disease. Hateful thoughts do enormous harm to your system. Worry, anger or hate can produce up to 1 pint of acid per minute in the body. So prolonged negative thoughts create a tremendous chemical imbalance in the body. Approaching problems with a calm and collected attitude will do wonders for your physical and mental wellbeing.

EATING

Eating is the favorite pastime of many, and the downfall of some. Nutritional imbalances play a large part in the originating causes of disease. Devitalized foods, such as cane sugar, white flour and foods with chemical additives cannot supply the proper amount of amino acids which nourish every cell in the body. Here are some informative hints on how to enjoy your food and derive more benefit from it by allowing your body to function at its best during the processes of digestion and assimilation.

Chewing

When you sit down to eat, make sure that you have plenty of time to relax and enjoy your meal, and that you are hungry! If you have only five minutes to "grab a bite to eat," skip the meal and sip a glass of juice or water instead. Wait until you have plenty of time to eat without swallowing your food whole. Gulping food or liquids does a tremendous disservice to your stomach and may result in headaches, stomachaches, gas and constipation. The hurried eater also loses part of the benefits of the vitamins and minerals in his or her food, as the digestive system is unable to continue functioning properly when the first step, mastication, is slighted. Saliva, secreted by the salivary glands, breaks down the starches and sugars in food and prepares them for the gastric juices in the stomach. Hastily eaten food misses the primary digestive process that depends upon thorough chewing and grinding in the mouth.

Overeating

Overeating creates problems throughout the system. A great many Americans suffer from distended colons, one of the results of overindulgence. Many of us, particularly in this country, feel a need to overeat because of the quality of the foods that we consume. When we eat devitalized foods the body is left with a feeling of dissatisfaction and sends signals to the brain that you are still hungry. When the proper foods are eaten, after a certain period of adjustment, the body will feel satisfied on far less. If you will eat only what you need, your body will not have to work so hard, and you will be freer of headaches and feelings of sluggishness.

Fruits and Vegetables

Fruits and vegetables eaten together or fruits eaten with other fruits may wipe out the nutritional benefits of both! Each fruit contains a different type of acid, and when one fruit is combined with another, the stomach becomes a battleground of acids. Consequently, fewer vitamins and minerals can be assimilated effectively by the system. Each day choose one type of fruit and eat as much of it as you like, but wait until the next day to have another. Eating combinations of fruits is sometimes responsible for little bumps on the ends of the fingers. This is due to the concentration of acids in conflict.

Fruits should never be eaten with vegetables. Vegetables may be eaten in any and all combinations without loss of benefits, but not within an hour of eating fruit. Occasionally you may wish to cheat and enjoy orange sauce on duck with asparagus, but fruit salads with dinner can create havoc in your stomach.

Save Your Stomach in the Morning

The first thing your body needs in the morning is fruit or fruit juice. The remains of last night's dinner may not yet be out of the stomach and the juice will help to clean out this food and prepare your stomach for today's food. Coffee and other strong acidic substances, when taken first thing in the morning, meet the undigested food creating an explosion of gases. Fresh fruit or fruit juice will stimulate the digestive processes and give your body a good start on the day. Orange juice may contain too much fruit sugar and tomato juice too much acid, but any type of juice you prefer is fine. You may eat or drink any type of fruit or fruit juice and have as much of it as you like, but wait at least one-half hour before eating anything else. If you start the day this way, you will find yourself more cheerful in the mornings and ready to tackle the day's activities.

Drinking

Drinking with meals can cause indigestion and gas. Food misses the salivary treatment when it is washed down with a drink. The food, then, must be broken down in the stomach, where it collides with the liquid and creates chaos. Drinking should be completed at least one-half hour before meals, and preferably one hour. This rule applies to water, wine, milk and all other liquids. The same time interval should be observed before drinking after a meal as well. Chronic stomach problems will often clear up within a week if this routine is observed faithfully.

You are wasting your body's energy if you gulp your food or liquids. Gulped liquids rush through the system, and your body does not have time to replenish and cleanse its cells. Sipping gives you the full benefit of the drink. Ideally, it should take you an hour to sip eight ounces of water and your body needs at least 24 ounces of water a day in addition to juices and herbal teas. When you drink the necessary amount of liquids, your body feels hungry less often as your cells will no longer be screaming for nourishment. Two-thirds of the body is made up of water. The body uses water to flush out used dead cells, toxins, and other wastes. All the body organs will suffer if proper amounts of water are not supplied. The kidneys, particularly, need water to function properly and when toxins cannot be flushed out by the kidneys, lower back pain can result.

Ice cold drinks can retard digestion and shock the stomach, especially after exercise. So try to drink all liquids at room temperature.

EXERCISE

Physical exercise facilitates proper digestion and, when lacking, causes clogging in both the digestive tract and the glandular system. Exercise should be part of your daily routine, and need not be strenuous or inconvenient. Swimming, dancing, walking and simply stretching will stimulate the body and help to relax tensions.

CHAPTER 2

GUIDES TO PREPARATION

GUIDES TO PREPARATION

Mother Nature has provided us with a natural remedy for almost any disease or malfunction, but you will benefit far more from her provisions if you know how to properly prepare your treatments. For the best results, follow the instructions given with each treatment, at least until you are familiar with its effects and results. Do not use herbal treatments while taking a chemical medication.

Because each of us is unique, some of us will respond better to one treatment and some to another. There are often many treatments given for one disease and you may use the one you prefer. I have marked the remedies which I find most effective with a ☆.

Do not expect an ailment of fifteen years to disappear overnight. On the other hand, once an ailment has been effectively treated herbally, there is little chance of recurrence as the herbs stimulate the body's production and protection mechanisms.

Herbs can be grown both indoors and outdoors, or may be purchased from various stores and suppliers, some of which are listed in the appendices. It is always best to use organically grown herbs. Harvest home grown or wild herbs with a wooden handled knife and, if possible, harvest when the sun is in the astrological sign of the herb. Herbs keep best in tightly sealed glass or ceramic containers and should not be exposed to direct sunlight or drastic temperature changes. Herbs that are grown, harvested and stored properly are more potent. Herbs also lose strength with age and should be discarded after 12-15 months, depending on the herb.

When preparing a treatment, make sure that you are using the correct part of the plant. The flowers, stems, leaves and roots of a plant may each have different properties, and where this is so, specific parts of the plant have been designated as the most useful. Herbal treatments are quite safe if directions are followed. Excesses, however, may reduce the efficiency of the treatment.

Do not use aluminum utensils, pots, pans or storage containers for any food related use. When water or food comes in contact with aluminum it undergoes a chemical change and picks up tiny particles of aluminum which accumulate in the liver, spleen and kidneys. Needless to say, aluminum should never be used, even for your pet's dishes.

TEAS

Herbs are usually taken in teas prepared in the following way. Place the tea or herb in a ceramic or glass container, pour boiling water over it, and allow to steep. Generally teas are made with a ratio of 1 teaspoon herb to 1 cup boiling water. Unless a recipe specifically instructs, do not boil the herb with the water as that can destroy the beneficial characteristics of the herb. Also, as a general rule, do not combine more than three herbs. If a particular tea seems bitter, you may add honey, but don't add sugar as it lessens the useful properties of the herb and also depletes body reserves of vitamins and minerals. Pure honey, on the other hand, is a natural sweetener which also contains valuable nutrients.

POULTICES

Poultices are useful for sprains, ruptures, drawing out infections, tension and swelling, and for drawing together cuts and broken bones. Poultices are most effective when made of fresh, organically grown fruits, vegetables or leaves which are grated, chopped, or crushed as directed. The herb is then wrapped in a clean, well-woven, non-irritating fabric such as muslin or cotton, and applied externally. In some cases, such as whiplash, it is best to use a cloth of pure silk, or silk mixture such as a scarf. As a last resort, paper towels may be used for poultices which are to be used for no more than 10 or 15 minutes. However, colored or recycled paper towels may contain impurities which will interfere with the healing process.

Poultices should be slightly damp and may be covered with a plastic bag to hold in the moisture. The poultice should be changed when dry or every 3-5 hours depending upon severity of the condition. Each time the poultice is changed, replace the cloth with a clean one.

If fresh herbs are not available, use dried herbs and pour boiling water over the herb to soften it before placing the herb inside the cloth.

Comfrey poultices are the most frequently used and are very simply made. Cut a piece of cloth twice as large as the area you wish to cover and use a freshly picked comfrey leaf. Wash the leaf in cool water and crush it in your hand. Spread the leaf on one side of the cloth, fold over the other half, and apply to affected part of the body (see diagram 2). Do not place the comfrey leaf directly against the skin as the leaf fuzz will irritate the skin. If the poultice is made with comfrey root or dried leaves, pour boiling water over the herb to soften and then use the strained root or leaves in the poultice and drink the resulting tea.

YOUR HOME MEDICINE CHEST

Your medicine cabinet need only contain the following items: garlic, alfalfa, comfrey, aloe vera and lemon. With these articles you can effectively treat almost every disease or condition. Garlic has been nicknamed the "body cleanser" as it can clean the entire blood system in less than an hour. Garlic also contains many nutrients. Alfalfa helps oxidize the blood, fight infection, and build up the body's resistance to disease. Comfrey, also known as knitbone, can be used for pulling cuts together, relieving swelling, dissolving internal growths, and drawing broken bones back into place. Comfrey has also been used to repair ruptured hernias in less than two weeks. Aloe vera is a form of cactus with wonderful medicinal properties. It soothes burns, relieves toothaches, helps heal cuts and bruises, and can be used for chapped lips and

13

rough skin. Lemon juice is the most antiseptic liquid known to man, more effective than rubbing alcohol or peroxide. Lemon juice soothes itchy bites, skin rashes, and when taken internally with water, helps cleanse, tone and relax the entire system. In addition, one drop lemon juice in an eye cup of warm water is a refreshing bath for the eyes. With these herbs on hand, you are well prepared to deal effectively with any emergency.

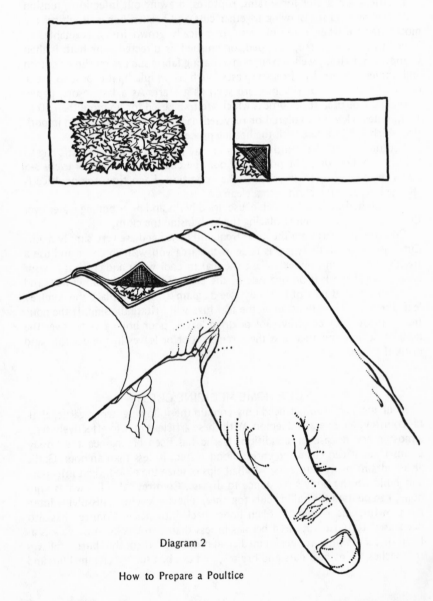

Diagram 2

How to Prepare a Poultice

CHAPTER 3

REMEDIES

ARTHRITIS, BURSITIS AND RHEUMATISM

These common diseases are caused by an over acid condition and are referred to by various names depending upon their severity and which parts of the body are affected. Arthritis, rheumatism and bursitis may all be regarded as "acidosis", and a treatment recommended for one of these diseases will be helpful for any of the other.

Excess acid in the body usually settles in the joints, causing inflammation and pain. In addition, this excess acid inhibits the production of natural cortisone in the body which feeds the adrenal glands and helps the body metabolize proteins.

The first step towards correcting acidosis is to eat only low acid or acid absorbing foods. Eliminate all sugars, white flour products, processed foods which contain chemicals, and high acid foods such as tomatoes and oranges. Also, avoid salt, vinegar, mustard, pepper, coffee, black teas, tobacco and alcohol. Potatoes and turnips are among the best foods to eat when suffering from acidosis as they are high in calcium, magnesium and vitamin D which help to absorb acids in the system and relieve stiffness in the joints. It is best to build your diet around low acid foods such as raw salads, fresh sprouts, pecans, brewer's yeast, wheat germ, raw vegetables (particularly potatoes and turnips), and low acid fruits to help stimulate the digestive system.

All Acidosis Conditions

To help restore the acid-alkaline balance in the body, combine the following ingredients and take three times a day, one hour before meals.

> 4 ounces tomato juice
> I teaspoon wheat germ
> I teaspoon yeast
> I teaspoon lecithin

☆Raw potatoes and turnips are excellent for acidosis. Eat as many as possible. Baked or boiled potatoes are also good, but should be eaten without topping (butter, sour cream, salt, etc.). If the potatoes are boiled, use the water as a soaking bath for hands and feet to relieve stiffness in the joints.

Alfalfa helps to relieve pain from acidosis. Eat fresh sprouts daily, take alfalfa tablets, or make alfalfa tea using I teaspoon herb to 1 cup boiling water. Drink 2-3 cups daily.

Rosemary, comfrey or nettles, taken in tea, help ease arthritic pain. Use ½ teaspoon powdered herb or leaves to 1 cup boiling water. Steep for 5 minutes and drink 2 cups per day.

Sage is helpful for both arthritis and rheumatism pain. Take 1 ounce sage (preferably white sage) to 1½ pints water. Simmer together for 20 minutes and take ½ cup when needed.

Cod liver oil helps relax and strengthen the joints when used daily. It also helps reduce popping noises of the joints. Apply externally.

Corn silk tea helps relieve arthritis pain and reduce acidic conditions in the body. Use only fresh corn silk in tea using 1 teaspoon herb to 1 cup boiling water. Drink when needed.

Parseley tea helps reduce acidosis pain. Use 1 quart boiling water and 1 cup packed parsley. Steep together for 15 minutes, strain and refrigerate. Use ½ cup as needed for pain.

Alehoof (ground ivy) is good for reducing arthritis pain. Use 1 teaspoon to 1 cup boiling water and take 2 cups per day. Crushed ivy leaves may be applied to swollen, painful joints to help relieve those conditions and draw out acids.

A canvas bag filled with oatstraw or with the hay chaff from a horse trough will help relieve stiff limbs when used in the bath. Drinking oatstraw tea (1 teaspoon oatstraw to 1 cup boiling water) helps internally.

Fresh string beans help acidosis because they contain vitamins A, B_1, B_2 and C. Eat daily or drink the bean juice freely.

Cherries and cherry juice help the body eliminate acids and take the bumps out of the knuckles. Take cherries or juice frequently every day for four days, stop for four days, and repeat.

White grape juice helps absorb the acid in the system. Drink 2-3 glasses daily.

To soothe aching muscles, combine the ingredients below and drink three times a day before meals.

    ½ tablespoon alfalfa powder
    1 tablespoon unfiltered honey
    1 tablespoon cider vinegar
    8 ounces water

Wintergreen oil rubbed into the affected joints will help relieve stiffness.

For neuritis, the following preparation is recommended. Combine the herbs and take 1-2 tablespoons of the mixture in 1 cup boiling water, steep for several minutes and strain. Drink 1 cup cooled mixture ½ hour before each meal.

    1 ounce lavender flowers
    1 ounce primrose
    1 ounce St. John's wort
    1 ounce blessed thistle
    1 ounce balm leaves
    2 ounces peppermint leaves
    3 ounces valerian root

Vitamin C supplements are good for all acidosis conditions. Take 100-1,000 milligrams daily when needed.

For gout and rheumatism use birthwort root which helps cleanse the stomach and lungs of phlegm. Use ½ ounce powdered root to 1 pint boiling water and drink 2-3 cups per day.

Combine the following ingredients and rub the liniment into affected areas for pain.

    ¼ teaspoon mustard oil
    ¼ teaspoon rosemary oil
    ¼ teaspoon cajeput oil
    ½ teaspoon mezereum bark
    1 teaspoon capsicum
    1 teaspoon wintergreen oil
    4 teaspoons cottonseed oil
    6 ounces turpentine oil
    3 ounce gum camphor

For rheumatoid arthritis, 600 mg of vitamins C and P (hesperidin) daily help improve the capillary condition.

Thuja, used externally, helps soothe arthritis pain. Use the leaves and twigs of thuja plant boiled with lard to make a salve. Apply externally when needed.

Combine 1 pound rosemary leaves with 1½ pounds lard and 2 ounces of beeswax and place in a large ceramic pot in a hot oven for 3 hours. This process will yield a salve which will help relieve arthritis pain. Strain the salve and apply externally to effected parts.

Lucerne herb, in powdered form, mixed with cider vinegar and honey makes a salve for severe arthritis. Use 1 teaspoon of each in a little water. Also use 1 ounce of the powder in 1 pint boiling water to make a tea. Steep 5 minutes, strain and drink 3 cups per day.

Gout

Gout signals the onset of arthritis and usually begins in the big toe. Corns and calluses which drain the fluid from the joints can contribute to this condition and should be taken care of immediately (see Skin section). In addition, the big toe should be rotated clockwise and counter-clockwise daily in order to help restore circulation.

Plaintain root, powdered or fresh, mixed with lard and spread onto a piece of leather and applied to the toe helps to draw out the acid.

Sarsaparilla, used 1 teaspoon to 1 cup boiling water and steeped for several minutes, helps gout. Take ½ cup three times a day for several months or until the condition clears.

Goutweed helps relieve pain in the joints. Use the herb in tea (1 teaspoon to 1 cup boiling water) or as a poultice applied to the affected parts.

Chives are a good food to eat to help reduce acidity in the system and relieve pain. The chives may also be made into a tea and taken daily.

Jasmine oil helps relieve pain and swelling of the joints due to acidosis.

Dandelion tea, which helps circulation, stimulates the red blood cells and helps flush excess acid from the system. Use 1 teaspoon dandelion root or leaves in 1 cup boiling water. Steep 5-10 minutes and drink 2-3 cups per day or when needed.

BACKACHES

Many people suffer from back pain. If any vertebrae or your pelvis is out of alignment, you should see a naturopath, osteopath, or chiropracter. He or she will be able to re-align your vertebrae or reposition your pelvis. Occasionally a negative mental state will cause pain in the back. Dr. Jackson says that "burden bearing thoughts" can help create backache. If this is the case, a positive outlook should bring relief. The lower back, or lumbar region, can become painful if you are not drinking enough water. If you do not take the time to drink sufficient fluids, the kidneys will not function properly and the resultant toxicity can cause pain.

Make sure you are drinking enough fluids (sipping not gulping!). Sip at least three 8 ounce glasses of water per day in addition to herbal teas and juices.

Massage the feet along the instep to help increase the circulation in the back and relax tension which may be concentrated there.

Dried Boston ivy is helpful for backaches. Use in tea, make with 1 ounce herb in 1 quart boiling water and allowed to cool. Drink 2-3 cups per day for six weeks to two months.

A poultice of bacon fat applied externally to the back will help to draw out pain.

BRAIN

All diseases of the brain, from insomnia to psychosis, can be treated with herbs, counseling and a healthy mental attitude. Many severe emotional disturbances originate from prolonged vitamin and mineral deficiencies. The brain requires plenty of lecithin, calcium, phosphorus and vitamins B and C. but without enough of any nutrient, the brain will suffer. Adequate daily exercise and a cheerful disposition will help to revitalize the brain and keep it healthy.

All Brain Malfunctions
Lecithin is needed by the brain in order to function properly, and it is recommended for all brain disorders. One tablespoon daily in liquid, granule or capsule form is sufficient. Lecithin is found in fertile eggs, soy products and, in small amounts, in all vegetables which have been vine ripened.

Phosphorus is essential to proper brain functioning. It is found in caraway seeds, apples and apple seeds, marygold, chipweed and horsetail herb. One or more of these herbs should be taken in tea or eaten daily.

Simple Tension and Nervousness
A daily warm bath, followed by a cool bath of salt water, helps relax the nervous system. Swimming in the ocean is always beneficial.

Dill strengthens the brain and calms tension in the stomach. Use 1 teaspoon dill to 1 cup boiling water. Drink several cups per day.

Juniper berries tone the nerves and strengthen the brain. Make a tea using 1 teaspoon berries to 1 cup boiling water. Steep for 5 minutes, strain and drink 2-3 cups per day.

Chia seeds help to calm the nerves. They may be made into tea or added to salads or cooking. To make in tea, use 1 teaspoon seeds to 1 cup boiling water. Drink 2-3 cups per day.

Restlessness may be caused by a need for calcium, magnesium and vitamin D. Turnips are a good source of these nutrients.

Basil is good for the nerves. Use 1 teaspoon in 1 pint water. Sip slowly during the day to calm tension.

Skullcap is a nervine and is also beneficial for the heart. It helps relax tension and promote sleep. Use 1 teaspoon in 1 cup boiling water, steep 3-5 minutes, and drink when needed.

Valerian helps calm the nerves. Use 1 teaspoon valerian to 1 cup boiling water and drink 2-3 cups per day.

Lemon juice and water sipped throughout the day will help tone the system and calm the nerves. Use the juice of 1 lemon in 8 ounces of water. Repeat up to six times.

Parseley tea is a mild sedative and contains nourishing vitamins and minerals. Use 1 teaspoon parseley to 1 cup boiling water or eat the fresh herb. Take as often as needed.

Before sleeping drink a mixture of ½ cup orange juice, ½ cup pineapple juice, and ¼ cup lemon juice. The combination will help to relax the body for sleep.

Garlic and onions are both powerful sedatives which soothe the brain. Use separately or mix together in tea and drink several cups per day.

Insomnia
☆For chronic sleeplessness, chop 1 clove garlic and place in a glass with just enough water to cover. Place a lid on the glass and allow the mixture to stand all day long. Just before bedtime fill the glass with water, as warm as you can drink, and sip slowly. Repeat this treatment daily for ten days to two weeks.

Sleeplessness is caused by an inability to relax. To promote relaxation, lie on the floor and slowly tense each part of the body beginning with the toes and working up the legs, torso, arms, neck and head. When the entire body is tense, release the tension altogether. This helps the body release tension.

Cucumbers are good for calming tension as they contain hormones and plenty of calcium.

Leaving salt out of the evening meal helps to promote sleep. The salt acts as stimulant to the system. Replacing the salt needs with dulse also gives a relaxing boost to the thyroid and glandular system.

Strawberry leaves make a tasty, relaxing tea. Use 1 teaspoon leaves to 1 cup boiling water. Sip warm tea slowly before bed.

Camomile tea helps to calm the nerves, revitalize the body, and stimulate the circulation in the hands and feet. Use 1 teaspoon camomile tea to 1 cup boiling water. Steep for 10 minutes, strain and drink before retiring.

Rosehips tea, taken before bed, helps facilitate sound sleep. The high amount of vitamin C in rosehips helps calm and soothe the nerves. Use 1 teaspoon hips to 1 cup boiling water, steep 10 minutes, strain and drink before bed.

A small amount of oil of cloves, taken with honey, helps to relax tense muscles.

One or two tablets of calcium (5-7 grains) in a glass of warm milk before bed will help you get to sleep.

One teaspoon nutmeg, taken in juice or milk before bed will help to relax tension and promote sleep.

To aid sleep, combine 4 tablespoons each skullcap, nerve root, and mint flowers with 1 quart water and boil mixture down to 1 pint. Drink 2 cups per day.

Carob leaf tea is relaxing to the entire nervous system. Use 1 teaspoon leaves to 1 cup boiling water and steep for 5 minutes. Take as needed for nervousness.

Lemon leaves, simmered for 20 minutes in 1½ cups of water, help relax tension and aid sleep. Drink before bed.

Raw or juiced celery is good for all types of nervousness and will help relax tension. Take daily when needed.

Oak groats are a good treatment for insomnia. Use 1 teaspoon powdered oat groats in 1 cup boiling water, steep for 3-5 minutes and sip slowly just before bedtime.

Make a tea with lungwort, using 1 teaspoon leaves to 1 cup boiling water. Take twice a day to help promote relaxation.

English lettuce helps to relax the nerves and promote sleep. English lettuce can be eaten raw in salads or juiced.

Hop flower tea will help relax the spinal column. Use 1 teaspoon hops flowers to 1 cup boiling water and drink several cups a day or when needed. Also, use a pillow stuffed with hops flowers to relax the body and promote sleep.

Brain Tonics

☆ Sage tea helps to revitalize the brain and improve concentration. Sage supplies oxygen to the cortex of the brain. Use 1 teaspoon sage to 1 cup boiling water and steep 3-5 minutes. Drink freely.

Mugwort and rosemary help to relieve mental fatigue and forgetfulness. Use 1 teaspoon of the combined herbs to 1 cup boiling water. Drink 3 cups per day.

Yerba mate will help stimulate the intellect and the body and tone the intestinal tract. Yerba mate is high in vitamin C, magnesium, silica and phosphates which feed the system. Use 1 teaspoon yerba mate to 1 cup boiling water and drink 3 cups per day.

Camomile stimulates the brain and helps to dispel weariness. Use 1 teaspoon camomile flowers to 1 cup boiling water and drink freely.

Dissolve ½ teaspoon barley in 2 cups boiling water, steep for 10 minutes, and take daily to help strengthen the brain.

Combine ½ cup apricot juice, 1 teaspoon lemon juice, 1 pinch kelp, 1 fertile egg yolk, and 1½ cups soy or goat milk. Blend the ingredients for 5 minutes and sip slowly. This mixture contains iron, vitamin C and many other nutrients which act as a tonic for the brain cells.

Dolomite (calcium and magnesium) aids the memory processes. Take 2-4 tablets per day. Each tablet contains approximately 125 mg. calcium and 75 mg. of magnesium.

Epilepsy

Epilepsy is caused by toxemia, or excess toxins in the system. This disease is characterized by nervous spasms and convulsions called seizures. When the body goes into convulsions, the seizure has already occurred within the brain. The body reacts to the seizure with a rush of adrenalin which, added to the excess toxins already in the blood, causes the nervous reaction of convulsion. At this point, the more blood you can divert to the brain to ease the shock and eliminate the excess adrenalin, the sooner the convulsions will cease. To help control seizures, place a belt around each leg between the knee and thigh and pull it tight (see diagram 3). Leave the belts in place for 1-2 minutes and release. This procedure will divert the blood flow to the upper part of the body, particularly the brain, and help to shorten the muscle spasms. Another way to help reduce a seizure is to step firmly on the patient's little finger of either hand. During all seizures take care to protect the patient from harm. After a seizure have the patient breathe fresh air and move around to stimulate circulation and minimize the aftereffects of the seizure.

Epileptics should be sure that they are getting plenty of B-complex vitamins and that they are not deficient in zinc. Dolomite (calcium and magnesium) and lecithin are also helpful when treating epilepsy.

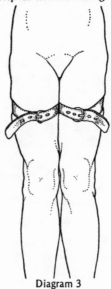

Diagram 3

Dittony is one of the best treatments for epilepsy. When taken daily for 6 months or more, dittony has been known to control seizures and gradually help stop them altogether. Use 1 teaspoon dittony in 1 cup boiling water and steep for 5 minutes. Take 1 tablespoon of the tea three times a day. During this treatment abstain from all meats except fish or poultry and take no chemicals into the body. Continue treatment whether seizures occur or not.

Cinquefoil is a good treatment for epilepsy and other diseases of the brain. Cinquefoil tea helps to remove poisons and congestion from any part of the body. Use 1 teaspoon of the root to 1 cup boiling water and take 2-3 cups per day. Continue for six months to two years or until all symptoms are gone.

Snakeroot is a good treatment for epilepsy because it is an anti-spasmodic herb. Use ½ ounce powdered plant to 1 pint boiling water. Take 3 cups per day.

Use 1 teaspoon valerian herb to 1 cup boiling water for epilepsy. Drink 2-3 cups per day.

Basswood is a good treatment for epilepsy. Use 1 teaspoon basswood in 1 cup boiling water, steep 3-5 minutes, and take ½ cup four times a day.

Calamint will promote recovery from all brain ailments. Use 1 teaspoon of the leaves and flowers in 1 cup boiling water and drink two cups per day.

Insanity

American mandrake sap can be used to treat all forms of insanity. Take ½ teaspoon of the fresh sap daily or use 1 teaspoon mandrake plant in 1 cup boiling water to make a tea. Drink 3 cups of the tea daily. Continue as necessary.

Holly seeds help strengthen the memory and are a useful treatment for all types of insanity. Make a tea using ½ teaspoon holly seeds to 1 cup boiling water. Drink 3 cups per day.

Make a tea using 1 teaspoon powdered vervain plant to 1 cup boiling water. Drink 1 cup every hour to treat all types of insanity.

Snakeroot tea is a good treatment for all mental disorders. This bitter herb will help cleanse the system of poisons. Use 1 teaspoon root to 1 cup boiling water or take an equivalent amount in capsule form.

Carrot seed tea helps in the treatment of all mental disorders by relaxing tension. Use 1 teaspoon seeds in 1 cup boiling water. Drink 2-3 cups per day.

Depression and Restlessness

Chronic melancholy or depression may be caused by deficiencies of vitamins C and E. See the Appendices for sources of these vitamins and eat daily.

If the spleen is not producing enough red blood cells, the subsequent lack of oxygen can cause depression. To stimulate the spleen, place 4 ounces hawthorne, 1 ounce cardamon, 1 ounce saffron, and ½ cup each balm and red sage in a burlap sack. Pour two quarts of boiling water onto the herbs and allow the mixture to steep for 24 hours. Then add 4 ounces of natural honey to the strained liquid and drink 1-2 cups when depressed.

Balm and ground ivy will help to restore the spirits. Make a tea using 1 teaspoon of the combined herbs to 1 cup boiling water. Sweeten with honey to taste and drink when needed.

Mayflowers will help to relieve nervous depression, restlessness and general pessimism. Use 1 teaspoon of the fresh plant to 1 cup boiling water. Take two cups per day.

Fit root helps to relieve restlessness and spasms. Use 1 teaspoon powdered fit root to 1 cup boiling water. Steep for 20 minutes and drink 2 cups per day.

Dodder is a good herb for the treatment of hypochondria. Make a tea using 1 teaspoon dodder to 1 cup boiling water. Drink 3 cups per day until condition clears.

Balm leaves help to restore the spirits. Make a tea using ½ teaspoon leaves to 1 cup boiling water. Drink 3 cups per day.

Myrrh, when burned as incense, will clear away negative energy. When taken as a tea, it will lift the spirits. Use ½ teaspoon powdered myrrh to 1 cup boiling water and drink 1-2 cups per day.

Passion flower is a good treatment for hysteria and will relax tension in the nervous system. Use 1 teaspoon of the herb to 1 cup boiling water and drink 2 cups per day.

Peppermint tea will help to relieve moodiness and relax the heart. Use 1 heaping teaspoon mint leaves in 1 cup boiling water. Drink freely.

A tea made of peppermint, catnip, rue and wood betony will help to clear obstructions in the system and relieve dizzyness. Use 1 teaspoon of the combined herbs to 1 cup boiling water. Drink early in the day.

Schizophrenia
Drink several glasses a day of carrot juice mixed with sage to help control schizophrenia. This combination will help to reduce the nervous tension and strengthen the brain. To keep the system clean and functional, eat only raw vegetables, fish or poultry and plenty of fruit. Do not eat red meats, sugar products or processed foods.

Manic Depression
Manic episodes may be controlled by giving the patient grapefruit sections with raw honey. This treatment will calm the nerves and supply the body with vitamin C and pantothenic acid. Manic Depressives should follow the diet recommended above, adding plenty of fresh vegetable juices.

The remedies recommended in the Depression and Restlessness section will also be helpful for manic depression.

Autism
Autistic children should be given plenty of fresh, raw vegetables, fruits and fresh juices. Do not let the autistic child eat any processed foods or foods containing chemical additives or colorings. The autistic child may be calmed by placing the hand on the back of the neck which helps to re-orient the child to surrounding energy. Sage tea will help to strengthen the brain and relax fear and tension. Use 1 teaspoon sage to 1 cup boiling water and sweeten with honey. Drink 3 or more cups per day.

Alcoholism
Alcohol destroys calcium, magnesium, iron and all vitamins, particularly vitamins B and D. Raw honey will supply some of these nutrients and the appendices give sources for replenishing the vitamins and minerals.

Delirium tremens (DT's) should be treated with bugle. This herb is a mild sedative and will help to control hallucinations. Use 1 teaspoon powdered bugle to 1 cup boiling water and drink 3 cups per day or take 5 grains daily in capsule form.

Angelica root or leaves will help to destroy the desire for alcohol. Use 1 teaspoon of this herb to 1 cup boiling water. Drink 3 cups per day.

Senility
Senility is not an incurable or unavoidable disease. The symptoms of senility are caused by vitamin and mineral deficiencies in the system. As the body ages more calcium is needed to keep the bones firm, the nervous system requires more vitamin C, and more potassium is needed to maintain muscle strength. An abscence of any vitamin or mineral will inhibit proper functioning of the aging system. Be sure a well balanced diet is followed. See the appendix for lists of foods high in these nutrients.

Sage tea will help to stop trembling of the limbs. Use 1 teaspoon sage to 1 cup boiling water and drink freely. This tea will also help to strengthen the brain and memory.

Brain Damage
Masterwort herb will stimulate the activity of the organs and help to reduce paralysis caused by hemorrhaging of the brain or spinal column. Use 1 ounce masterwort root to 1 pint boiling water and drink ½ cup three times a day.

Black walnut hull tea will help to restore damaged cells in the brain. Use 1 teaspoon hulls to 1 cup boiling water and steep for 10-15 minutes. Slowly sip three cups per day.

Mongolism may be caused by improper assimilation of vitamins and minerals by the mother during pregnancy. The child should be given vitamins B, C, and E daily in food and in supplemental form to help stimulate normal growth.

Sage tea is an excellent treatment for mental retardation as it will increase the circulation to the brain and feed the cortex. Use 1 teaspoon sage to 1 cup boiling water and drink 3-5 cups per day for 6 months to 1 year. Improvement should be obvious and treatment should be continued as needed.

CANCER, TUMORS AND CYSTS

Cancer is one of the most dread diseases, but it can be controlled and even eliminated with the proper mental attitude and diet. Most cancers begin in the same way: an organ or section of the circulatory system becomes clogged with impurities which stagnate and begin to reproduce. To alleviate the condition, the blood stream and all of the organs must be thoroughly cleansed. If you are told you have cancer, immediately exclude from the diet all protein foods such as meat, eggs, beans, lentils, and cheese. This will "starve" the reproducing cells. Eat only raw fruits, vegetables and juices as these foods will cleanse the system and allow the body to fight the cancer. If the treatment is to be successful, the entire system must be kept free of all obstructions and the blood stream must be kept pure.

Internal and External Cancers
☆Make the following juices fresh daily and, in addition, drink at least three 8-ounce glasses of water. Eat no other foods. This diet will supply the body with all the nutrients needed, but will not support the cancerous growths.

On day one, drink 10 ounces carrot juice and 6 ounces spinach juice.

On day two, drink 3 ounces spinach juice, 2 ounces parsley juice, 4 ounces celery juice and 7 ounces carrot juice.

On day three, drink 3 ounces each of beet and cucumber juice, and 10 ounces carrot juice.

On day four, drink 2 ounces coconut juice, 3 ounces beet juice, and 11 ounces carrot juice.

On day five, drink 1 pint spinach juice.

On day six, drink 2 ounces parsley juice, 5 ounces celery juice, and 9 ounces carrot juice.

On day seven, drink 12 ounces carrot juice and 4 ounces parsley juice.

On day eight, start the diet over again with day one and continue in sequence until condition is completely cleared.

Watercress helps supply vitamins and nutrients to the system and helps to clear cancerous growths. Eat in salad or drink watercress juice daily.

Horsetail herb is a good treatment for both internal and external cancers. Use 2 large handfuls in 1 quart boiling water, steep for 10 minutes and strain. Add honey, if needed, and drink 4-5 cups daily.

Oatstraw helps rebuild the minerals in the system. A cloth soaked in oatstraw tea and placed on the skin will help to stop decay and control engorgement. Make a tea using 2 large handfuls of oatstraw to 1 quart boiling water. Let steep for 10 minutes, strain, and apply externally. In addition, drink 4-5 cups per day.

To reduce the offensive odor of cancerous decay, use powdered charcoal and yeast in a poultice over the affected areas. Change the poultice often and burn the cloth and residue.

Grated raw carrot, made into a poultice, will help soothe inflammation and reduce odor. Cooked, raw, and juiced carrots are beneficial for all types of cancer because of the nutrients they contain. If carrots are cooked, be sure to drink the liquid in which they cook.

Grapes help to control cancer as they contain cell salts which nourish the blood system. A diet of nothing but grapes may be eaten for three months. Take care to drink only distilled water, at least one cup per hour. When using the grape diet, eat the seeds, skins and meat of the grape.

Comfrey leaves, in a poultice, will help to control cancerous growths and, when combined with comfrey tea, will help to clean out the system. Drink 5 or more cups of comfrey tea per day and change the poultices at least 3 times a day.

To help heal cancerous growths, use ½ pound red clover to 1 pint water. Simmer the mixture until it is reduced to a syrup. Watch carefully to prevent burning. Spread this syrup onto a cloth and apply daily. Repeat until completely cleared.

A poultice of crushed, fresh cranberries will raise pustules on the cancerous skin. This "blistering" is the cancerous tissue being drawn out of the body. Changing the poultice at least three times a day, gently wipe the area with a clean, sterile cloth and re-apply poultice. Continue until pustules no longer appear.

Crush fresh blue or white violet leaves and use in a poultice to help draw out cancerous growths. Also, make a tea of the leaves and take internally. Use 1 teaspoon leaves to 1 cup boiling water and drink 3-5 cups per day.

Poultices should be used directly over the effected external area and over the diseased internal area. During all stages of treatment, drink only distilled water and eat plenty of roughage foods. A diet consisting of raw fruit for one meal, raw vegetables for the next, then fruit again, etc. is the best to follow. Other than fruits, vegetables, and juices, eat one slice of sourdough bread each day. Continue the diet until all growths are gone and the body has returned to functioning properly.

Sarcoidosis, a form of cancer of the lungs, may be treated by using the cranberry poultice regimen given before along with daily breathing exercises. Fill the lungs with air from the abdomen up through the chest. This will help to strengthen the lungs and insure an adequate supply of oxygen.

Brain Tumors

Tumors in the brain may be drawn out by placing a poultice of fresh grape juice at the nape of the neck. This poultice should be changed when dry and treatment should be continued until the growth is gone. Comfrey tea and plenty of raw juices will help to facilitate this process.

Leukemia

Leukemia is a form of cancer which destroys the marrow of the bones. The above diets may be used and cranberry juice should be added. The liver, spleen, and pancreas must be kept clean and functional so that new blood cells can be produced as quickly as they are needed.

Cysts

Cysts anywhere in the body may be treated with comfrey tea. This tea should be drunk 5 or more times a day to help the healing process and a comfrey poultice should be placed on the skin outside the affected area.

The juice diet given at the beginning of this section is another helpful way to treat cysts of the internal organs. Follow the diet for at least 10 days to insure that the cysts are dissolved.

Dolomite and garlic pearlies (garlic oil in capsules) are helpful for dissolving cysts. Take in tablet form or eat in foods.

CHRONIC AND DEGENERATIVE DISEASE

Most degenerative diseases, including multiple sclerosis (MS), muscular dystrophy and palsy are caused by a form of malnutrition which results from a continuous diet of devitalized and processed foods. Vitamin deficiencies from this type of a diet will result in the deteriorization of the myelin sheath which covers and protects the nerves. This break down of myelin causes a loss of resistance to infection, muscular spasms, and a gradual loss of control over the entire muscle system. Fatty acids contain vitamin F and this deficiency, coupled with deficiencies of vitamins B, C, and E as well as dolomite, will eventually cripple the body. To treat these diseases, the first step is to completely eliminate from the diet all processed foods, liquids and sugars. Brown rice contains many nourishing minerals and vitamins which can help rebuild the nervous system. The following remedies are also helpful.

Multiple Sclerosis and Muscular Dystrophy

Each day for one week take only fresh fruit juices, some raw goat milk and 1 slice of sourdough bread. Drink only one type of juice each day. During the second week, eat only raw fruit for one meal and raw vegetables for the next, then raw fruit again, etc. Eat many different kinds of fruits and vegetables to insure a proper supply of vitamins and minerals. Be sure to take only one type of fruit or fruit juice per day. Carrot, spinach, parseley and cucumber juices are helpful. Continue with 1 slice of sourdough bread per day.

Muscular dystrophy attacks the body in much the same way as multiple sclerosis. It usually begins from the same basic reasons. Muscular dystrophy must be treated with raw fruits and vegetables and lots of vitamin F. Apple pits contain large quantities of vitamin F, and alfalfa supplies vitamin F as well as A,B,C,K,P,G, and many minerals.

Fast for five days alternating fruit juice one day and vegetable juices the next. Thereafter, stay with a strict diet of raw fruit and vegetables for the next two weeks. Place an emphasis on keeping the system alkaline. After the first five days, add to the diet some sprouted wheat and 1 slice per day of sour dough bread. This diet will help to rebuild the nervous system and stimulate the metabolism. Smoking and drinking alcoholic beverages must be eliminated entirely. Also eliminate coffee, any form of sugar, and all white flour or bread products except the prescribed sourdough bread.

To make a tonic for degenerative diseases, cut up 1 pound unpeeled raw beets and cover with ¼ pound each brown sugar and natural honey. Allow mixture to stand for 48 hours. Take 1 ounce morning and evening every day until condition is completely cleared.

American century is a good herb to take while recovering from degenerative diseases as it helps to build up the body. Use 1 teaspoon of the herb to 1 cup boiling water and steep for ½ hour. Drink two cups of the cold tea per day.

Graves Disease (Parkinson's Disease)

Make a tea using 2 ounces speedwell to 1 pint boiling water. Steep for 5-10 minutes and take 1 ounce daily for Graves Disease.

Palsy

To treat palsy, use the tonic given above.

Sage tea helps to quiet the tremors of the limbs. Use 1 teaspoon sage to 1 cup boiling water and steep for 5-10 minutes. Sip slowly, 3-5 cups per day or as needed.

Five to six grains of black cohosh taken daily, will help to control involuntary spasms of palsy and St. Vitus dance disease.

Chickweed leaf ointment will help to stop the tremor of the limbs. Apply to the legs to treat varicose veins. Use 1 ounce chickweed leaves combined with 1 pound cocoa butter or paraffin. Warm until mixed and then allow to steep for several minutes. Apply to effected parts after it is cool enough.

Fit root is a good treatment for fainting and spasms of all kinds. Use 1 teaspoon fit root and 1 teaspoon fennel seed in 1 pint boiling water. Steep for 20 minutes and drink 1-2 cups per day.

Paralysis

Paralysis is caused by a block in the flow of blood to a particular organ or limb. Care should be taken to insure that the system is kept clean and functioning properly. Here are some herbs which help in the treatment of paralysis.

Paralysis of the tongue may be treated with ginger leaf tea. Use one or two leaves or 1 teaspoon dried leaves to 1 cup boiling water. Drink hot. Sip 2 cups per day.

Prickly ash is a good treatment for paralysis of the tongue and mouth. Use 1 ounce prickly ash bark or leaves to 1 pint boiling water, steep 15 minutes, and drink 3-4 cups per day.

Snakeroot will stimulate the system and help to remove blockages. Use ½-1 teaspoon snake root to 1 cup boiling water, steep 3 minutes and sweeten with honey. Take 1-3 cups per day.

Lecithin, which is contained in every cell in the brain and spinal column, can help to dissolve blockages which cause paralysis. Take 1 tablespoon in liquid, powder, granules, or capsule form daily.

Polio

To treat polio, take 600 mg each of vitamins C and P (hesperidin) per day until the capillary activity is improved. Vitamin P is found in the white part of the skin of all citrus fruits. Eat plenty of bioflavoids which are found in berries, currents, plums, apricots and lemons.

Green peppers are a rich source of vitamins and minerals and are very good for helping to treat polio.

Dropsy (Edema)

Dropsy is the condition of excessive water retention in the body. If not remedied, an extreme case of dropsy can literally drown the patient. Dropsy indicates that the kidneys, pancreas and liver are all malfunctioning. The sections dealing with diseases of these organs will give further information on specific treatments of the organs. Here are some general remedies for dropsy.

For Bright's disease and dropsy take queen of the meadow root tea. Use 1 teaspoon of the root to 1 cup boiling water, steep for 10 minutes, and drink ½ cup three times a day.

The inner bark of the white ash is a good treatment for dropsy. Steep 1 teaspoon bark in 1 cup boiling water for 30 minutes. Strain and drink ½ glass 4-5 times a day.

Juniper berries help the body to eliminate excess fluids. Use 5-7 berries to 1 pint boiling water. Steep for ½ hour, strain and take 1-2 ounces per day.

Yarrow flowers help to stimulate the eliminative processes. Use 1 teaspoon to 1 cup boiling water and steep for 5-10 minutes. Drink 4 cups per day.

Horseradish, freshly ground or eaten raw, will help the body to eliminate excess fluids. Eat ½ cupful daily.

Falling Sickness

Falling sickness is a form of epilepsy. Parseley, fennel, anise and caraway will help to stimulate the body and prevent falling sickness. Use the roots, seeds, and leaves of any of the above herbs, one herb at a time, mixing 1 ounce herb to 1 pint boiling water. Steep 5-10 minutes, strain and take 4 ounces liquid morning and evening. After taking the tea, do not eat or drink anything for at least 3 hours. In addition, see the Brain section for more information.

Meningitis

Meningitis is an illness of the fluid which surrounds and protects the brain. It can be treated by shaving the back of the head and immersing the back of the head in a bowl of epsom salts and warm water. This helps to draw out the inflammation. In addition, the patient should be given comfrey tea to drink. Make the tea using 1 teaspoon comfrey leaves to 1 cup boiling water. Steep 3-5 minutes, strain and drink freely. Use at least 5 cups of the tea per day to help strengthen the system and fight the infection.

Sciatica

The sciatic nerve runs from the heel of the foot up the legs and through the body. Massaging the back of the heel and up the entire leg can help to relieve the pain of sciatica.

Jasmine oil will help to soothe sciatic pain and the bark may be made into a tea. Use ½ teaspoon bark to 1 cup boiling water and steep for 3-5 minutes. Drink 1-2 cups per day as needed.

Vitamin D, taken with calcium and magnesium, will be assimilated properly by the body and help to ease sciatic pain.

To treat sciatica combine ½ cup darnel, ½ teaspoon honey and 1½ cups distilled water. Steep several minutes, strain and sip slowly, ½ cup at a time, during the day.

Rue is a good treatment for sciatic pain. Make a tea using 1 teaspoon rue to 1 cup boiling water. Steep 5 minutes, strain and drink 2-3 cups daily or when needed.

COUGHS AND COLDS

Sore throats, coughs and colds all indicate congestion in the system. Do not eat or drink any milk or milk products as they are acid and mucous forming. Goat or soy milk products may be substituted as these products are alkaline and non-mucous forming. To treat these conditions, you must clear the congestion in the body and a juice or other liquid diet for several days will help to clean the digestive tract and relieve the cold. Drinking a quart of fruit juice a day is a good way to build up body resistance and to prevent colds. Here are other ways of relieving these conditions.

Sore Throats

For sore throats, slowly roast a ripe lemon in the oven until it cracks open, and take 1 teaspoon of the juice with a little honey once every hour. This mixture is also good for hacking coughs.

To reduce swelling from sore throats, make a poultice using cudweed and cover with plastic. Change the poultice 2-3 times a day.

Make a tea using ½ teaspoon mouseroot in 1 cup boiling water to use as a gargle for mouth irritations. Gargle twice a day and drink the remaining tea.

Queen's delight and sundew herbs help to control coughing and laryngitis. Use 1 teaspoon of the herbs to 1 cup boiling water and drink 1 cup twice a day.

Mix 4 tablespoons of cider vinegar and 1 pint boiling water to make a good, antiseptic mouthwash. Gargle several times a day.

Sage tea is an excellent gargle for sore throats. Use morning and evening and when needed throughout the day. Use 1 teaspoon sage to 1 cup boiling water, steep several minutes, and strain. Drink remainder of the tea.

☆Gargle with diluted lemon juice one hour and black tea the next hour alternately all day to help clear sore throats and laryngitis. Do not drink the black non-herbal tea, but the tannic acid it contains is good for soothing the throat when used intermittently with the lemon and warm water.

Assesmart helps to clear up thrush (mouth ulcers) and is a soothing gargle for sore throats. Use 1 ounce leaves to 1 pint cold water. Drink 3 ounces when thirsty in place of water. As a gargle, use 3-5 times per day.

Garlic is a good treatment for colds and hacking coughs. Eat 1 bulb daily.

Balm tea helps to soothe the throat and strengthen the voice for singing. Use 1 teaspoon balm leaves to 1 cup boiling water, steep 3-5 minutes and add 1 teaspoon honey. Sip slowly, repeating as needed.

Cooked barley mixed with lemon and water helps to soothe sore throats. Use enough water to liquify the mixture and gargle when needed.

Bush honeysuckle made into a tea is a good gargle for sore throats. Use ¼ tea-spoon herb to 1 cup boiling water. Gargle several times a day.

Mix equal parts of yarrow, elderberry and peppermint and make into a tea using 1 teaspoon of the combined herbs to 1 cup boiling water. This tea helps cleanse the system of congestion and stimulate elimination, take freely at the first sign of a cold.

Pennyroyal tea is good for coughs and colds. Make the tea using 1 teaspoon pennyroyal leaves to 1 cup boiling water and drink several cups per day.

Avens herb is a good treatment for fever, colds and sore throats. Make a tea using 1 teaspoon herb to 1 pint boiling water. Drink 3 cups per day.

Clover tonic is good for all bronchial ailments and colds and it helps to build up the body's resistance to disease. Steep 1 teaspoon clover in 1 cup boiling water and drink often during the day.

Bayberry tea helps cleanse the throat of putrid substances. Use 1 teaspoon bayberry to 1 cup boiling water and steep for 30 minutes. Gargle often until the condition improves. Drink a pint of the lukewarm tea to throughly cleanse the stomach and help to restore normal mucous production.

For cankers in the mouth, mix ½ teaspoon each of barberry bark, bistort, and red raspberry leaves and pour 1 pint boiling water over the mixture. Steep 5-10 minutes and drink often until condition improves.

Thyme tea helps to prevent colds and infections. Use 1 teaspoon to 1 cup boiling water and drink freely throughout the day.

Comfrey tea, prepared using 1 teaspoon leaves to 1 cup boiling water, helps promote healing of colds and infection. Drink 4 or more cups per day.

Make a tea using 1 teaspoon St. John's wort to 1 cup boiling water. Drink and go to bed. The herb will induce perspiration and help to control coughing.

Angelica root is an expectorant and will help to control coughs, colds and all bronchial ailments. Use ¼ teaspoon root to 1 pint boiling water. Drink slowly, several cups per day.

Eat small amounts of grated horseradish mixed with honey to help control hoarseness.

For swollen throat glands, use a poultice of crushed ground ivy leaves. Cover the poultice with a piece of plastic to keep the heat in and change when dry.

A tea using 1 teaspoon of the bull rushes root to 1 cup boiling water helps control chronic coughs. Drink ½ cup three times a day.

Parsnips are a good treatment for shortness of breath and coughs. Use 1 teaspoon parsnip root to 1 cup boiling water and drink two cups per day.

Lungwort is a good treatment for coughs and to expel mucous. Boil 1 ounce of the dried leaves and 1 pint milk in a double boiler for 10 minutes. Other cooking processes will cause constipation. Sweeten with honey to taste and sip often to ease throat congestion.

American cowslip tea is a mucous expectorant which is useful for colds and chronic chest congestion. Use 1 teaspoon cowslip to 1 cup boiling water to make a tea. Steep 5-10 minutes and drink two cups per day.

Use the entire wild evening primrose plant to make a tea to treat coughs and colds. Use 1 teaspoon herb, cut into small pieces, in 1 cup boiling water. Drink the cold tea slowly throughout the day.

Ginger leaf tea will help to stop colds at the onset. Use 1 teaspoon ginger to 1 cup boiling water and drink hot, ½ cup at a time. Ginger warms the body and stimulates the circulation.

Dandelion tea helps to clear cold infections. Use 1 teaspoon dandelion greens to 1 cup boiling water and drink freely.

Monkshood is a good treatment for fevers, colds, coughs and to ease bronchial congestion. The powdered monkshood root mixed with egg white and applied to the chest, helps to draw out the congestion. Remove when dry and repeat if necessary.

Dill tea, used 1 teaspoon herb to 1 cup boiling water, is good for coughs. Drink two cups per day.

To help relieve colds and sniffles, press the juice of grated black horseradish and mix with up to ½ pound of honey. Take 2 tablespoons before each meal and one hour before bedtime.

Chervil is a good treatment for coughs. Make a tea using 1 teaspoon herb to 1 cup boiling water. Take 1 tablespoon three times a day.

Coltsfoot is a helpful remedy for colds and coughs. Use 1 teaspoon of the leaves to 1 cup boiling water and steep for ½ hour. Drink freely.

Cayenne is recommended for people who have been exposed to colds and as a treatment for already established colds. Take 5-20 grains in warm water or in capsule form. Do not exceed recommended dosage as excess cayenne can irritate the mucous membranes of the digestive tract.

Bloodroot is a mucous expectorant and is a good treatment for colds. Use 1/12 grain to 1 pint water. Take 1 teaspoon three times a day.

Pleurisy root is a good treatment for colds, flu, fever, asthma, and chest infections of all kinds. Use 1 teaspoon powdered root in 1 cup boiling water. Drink 4-5 cups per day.

Allergies and Hayfever

Allergic reactions are caused when the antigen production of the liver, pancreas and spleen exceed the normal production. This condition indicates a lack of vitamin C, calcium and magnesium. Sugars, and all sugar products further deplete these nutrients and milk and milk products clog the system. Allergies and hayfever conditions can be controlled by eliminating all nonnutricious foods from the diet and by building the body resistance to a level which can strengthen the system. Canned foods should be replaced with a diet of fresh fruits and vegetables and especially fruits with pits in them. Eat plenty of vitamin C rich foods such as apricots, peaches and cherries.

Red clover helps to build up the body resistance to allergies. Use 1 teaspoon clover blossoms to 1 cup boiling water and steep for 5-10 minutes. Drink 3-4 cups per day before coming in contact with allergy or hayfever causes. During the season, or if an attack occurs, double your intake of tea and take large amounts of vitamin C per hour. Rosehips supply the most easily assimilated sources of vitamin C.

Farum phos, a cell salt, is good for treating hayfever. Dissolve three of the small tablets on the tongue, every two hours for the first day, and thereafter, three times a day.

Licorice helps to build up resistance to allergens. Use 3 roots of licorice to 1 quart water. Boil together for 10 minutes, strain, and take 1 tablespoon 3 times per day every other day for a six day period.

Mononucleosis

Mono or, the kissing disease, is caused by a combination of nervous and physical exhaustion due to a lack of proper nutrients in the diet and an excess of stress. However, in the early stages, it may be contagious, hence its secondary name.

For mono, take 1 clove chopped garlic in 1 teaspoon olive oil first thing in the morning. Eat no food until the bowels move and repeat the next day. Take only vegetable juices for the next two days, particularly carrot, celery, spinach or parseley juice. Take apple or pumpkin juice for days three and four. Drink about 8 ounces of liquid each hour during these four days and repeat this diet until condition is cleared. This stimulates the entire system to eliminate the blockages caused by devitalized foods.

Asthma, Bronchitis and Chest Infections

☆ Blue violet leaf tea will help to dry out the moisture in the lungs which activates asthma attacks. Use 1 teaspoon leaves to 1 cup boiling water and drink two cups daily. Continue for several months to help completely dry the lungs.

Masterwort helps to control asthma by stimulating the activity of the lungs. Use 1 ounce masterwort to 1 pint boiling water and steep for 10 minutes. Take ½ cup three times a day.

Honeysuckle is a good treatment for asthmatic conditions. Use ½ teaspoon to 1 cup boiling water and take 1 cup 3-4 times a day.

Jerusalem artichokes contain vitamins A, B_1, B_2 and C and will nourish the lungs and help to relieve asthmatic conditions. Eat raw or in soups or salads.

Prickly ash helps to remove obstructions from the system and will help to clear the lungs. Use ½ teaspoon prickly ash to 1 pint boiling water. Drink 4 or more cups per day.

Apricots contain many nutrients which promote healing of lung conditions such as tuberculosis (TB), bronchitis, and asthma. Eat 3-6 apricots daily.

Vitamin E promotes healing of the lungs and helps to rebuild cells. Asthmatic sufferers should eat foods which are high in vitamin E and take supplements daily. Start with a low dosage and, over a period of several weeks, increase up to 1,200 i.u. per day.

Pennyroyal will help asthmatic congestion. Use 1 teaspoon leaves and flowers in 1 cup boiling water. Sweeten with honey to taste and take 1 teaspoon two times a day.

Yerba mate will help to control pain in the lungs and increase respiratory capacity. Use ½ teaspoon yerba mate to 1 cup boiling water and take 3-5 cups per day.

Cockleburr tea is a good treatment for asthma. Steep 2 handfuls in 1 quart of boiling water and drink 1 cup four times a day.

Two handfuls of wild plum bark steeped in a quart of boiling water helps to control asthma attacks. Take 1-2 cups daily.

To help sleep, asthmatics may sleep on a pillow stuffed with life everlasting herb.

Speedwell helps to eliminate obstructions in all parts of the body, including the lungs. Use 2 ounces speedwell to 1 pint boiling water and take ½ ounce per day.

For asthma, mix equal parts of garlic, ginseng, magnesium and vitamin C. Take ½ teaspoon of the combined mixture before each meal. This remedy is not recommended for women because of the use of the ginseng

Boil 3 licorice roots in 1 pint water and sip throughout the day for asthma.

To treat bronchial asthma, mix onions, honey and skunk cabbage or garlic. Steep mixture with enough water to make a tea and drink 1 cup daily.

Bronchial asthma sufferers should abstain from all meats, eggs, bread and milk products, as these products will create more mucous in the system.

Mix two tablespoons ground flax seeds with 1 pint boiling water, simmer for 2 or 3 minutes, strain and sip slowly. This tea helps clear out mucous from bronchial tubes and colds.

Vervain promotes perspiration which helps the body to expel phlegm and bronchial mucous. Use 1 teaspoon vervain and 1 cup boiling water to make a tea. Steep 3-5 minutes, strain and sip 1-2 cups per day. This herb works quickly.

White bryony helps to cleanse mucous from the lungs. It is useful for treating pneumonia, tonsilitis, glandular swelling and all bronchial ailments. Use 1 ounce powdered bryony to 1 pint boiling water and take 1 tablespoon morning and evening. Continue daily for up to six months or, as long as needed. Asthma and emphysema patients should not exceed the recommended dosage as the condition must be treated slowly to allow time for the lungs to replace diseased cells.

For bronchitis, mix ½ ounce each of hyssop, comfrey root and coltsfoot with 1 pint boiling water and steep for 10 minutes. Drink ½ cup twice a day. For severe conditions, take up to three cups per day.

For flu and bronchial ailments, use 1 teaspoon blue violet leaves to 1 cup boiling water. Steep for 2-3 minutes and sip slowly. Drink 2-3 cups daily to help remove mucous.

Fenugreek will help to expel phlegm and cleanse the kidneys. Use 1 teaspoon to 1 pint boiling water and drink ½ cup of the tea twice a day.

Vitamin A is helpful in all bronchial troubles. Fresh parseley, watercress and alfalfa are good sources of this vitamin.

Dry nettle leaves help to purify the blood and dissolve mucous in the lungs and glands. It is also used to cleanse the stomach of undigested food. Use 1 teaspoon leaves to 1 cup boiling water and drink ½ cup three times a day.

Mayflower herb is a good decongestant and will help to control mucous in the nasal cavity. Use 1 teaspoon of the herb to 1 cup boiling water and drink ½ cup three times a day.

To treat flu, colds, chest infections and malaria, bake a lemon in the oven until it splits open. Beat the lemon juice with 1 tablespoon grape brandy and 2 pinches of salt. After taking a hot bath, before retiring, drink the mixture and take 10 drops jaborandi in a cup of hot water. After 6 hours, sponge down and rub the body with oil.

Mullein flower tea is a good treatment for chest and bronchial ailments. Use 1 teaspoon flowers to 1 pint boiling water. Take 1 tablespoon three times a day to loosen phlegm.

Cooked barley mixed with lemon and water is a good treatment for bronchitis. Liquify the mixture in a blender and sip slowly.

To expel mucous, mix the juice of 1 spanish onion, 1 teaspoon salt, and ½ glass water and gargle. Drink fenugreek tea daily, and continue for several weeks until mucous is gone.

Dandelion is an effective blood cleanser and body purifier. It contains plenty of vitamin C which promotes healing of tuberculosis. Use 1 teaspoon herb to 1 cup boiling water and drink at least three cups per day.

Garlic is the most common blood purifier, one bulb per day will build resistance to tuberculosis and help to clear up the condition once contracted.

Apricots help to supply nutrients needed by TB patients. Eat 3-5 daily.

Horehound leaves are a good mucous expectorant. When this herb is boiled down to syrup form, it may be used to treat colds, coughs, asthma and TB. The tea may be used to promote perspiration and urination. Use 1 teaspoon horehound to 1 cup boiling water and steep for 5 minutes. Sip slowly over a period of several hours.

Sinusitis
Blue berries, carrots, and cucumbers are all good for stuffy sinuses. They may be eaten fresh or juiced.

Fresh ground ivy tea will help to relieve nasal congestion and stop headaches. Use 1 teaspoon ivy leaves to 1 cup boiling water. When cooled, sniff up the nose.

Take two tablets of garlic and parseley every four waking hours for six days. This helps to clear up chronic sinus trouble.

Mix chopped onions and garlic and eat to help soothe the mucous lining of the nose and sinuses. This treatment also kills any harmful bacteria in the nose and mouth.

Garlic helps to control nicotine poisoning and helps in the treatment of all respiratory infections including sinusitis. Take 1 bulb per day.

Pour a strong tea of mellilot herb over the head after washing the hair to help clear up sinus conditions.

To help soothe and clean the sinuses follow the diet listed below for four days. Thereafter, eat horseradish once a week with fish and rice. Be sure to take at least 3 eight ounce glasses of water per day and abstain from all milk and milk products.

On day one, drink 6 ounces spinach juice and 10 ounces carrot juice.

On day two, eat 1 pint horseradish with 1 whole lemon.

On day three, drink 10 ounces carrot juice, and 3 ounces each of beet and cucumber juice.

On day four, drink 1 pint carrot juice.

For all sinus conditions, massage underneath the big toe on both feet and each of the toes. Repeat daily.

Take a spoonful of honey with 2 drops of eucalyptus oil to help clear sinuses. Take just before retiring.

Vitamin A promotes healthy functioning of the nasal cavity, sinuses and the entire respiratory tract. A lack of vitamin A can lower resistance to infections in these areas. Eat plenty of chickweed, alfalfa and parseley to supply these nutrients.

Make an ointment using chickweed or archangel and lanolin. Use the herb in powder form. Apply the ointment to the face, let dry and repeat. This treatment helps shrunken sinuses become more pliable.

To clear the sinuses, take a warm bath and abstain from all milk products. Mix grated horseradish with lemon juice to make a thick sauce. Take 1 teaspoon of the mixture morning and evening to help clear nasal congestion. Do not eat or drink anything for 1 hour before or after taking the mixture.

Horehound leaves are a good mucous expectorant. Use 1 teaspoon leaves to 1 cup boiling water, steep and sip over a period of several hours. In addition, the syrup made from boiling the leaves and roots down helps to treat colds, coughs, asthma, sinusitis and tuberculosis. Take 1 teaspoon of the syrup daily until the condition is cleared.

Emphysema

Emphysema is a bronchial condition which is characterized by excess mucous in the lungs. Bryony and blue violet leaves are good for clearing this congestion. Use 1 ounce bryony powder to 1 pint boiling water and take 1 tablespoon twice a day. In severe cases, the dosage may be increased to three times a day. Do not exceed this dosage as the lungs must be cleared gradually in order to replace damaged cells. Use only white bryony and continue treatment for six months or more until condition is completely cleared.

Blue violet leaves are also good for emphysema. Use 1 teaspoon blue violet to 1 cup boiling water and steep for 2-3 minutes. Drink 2-3 cups per day.

Fever

☆To reduce fever, squeeze the juice from one grapefruit and put aside in the refrigerator. Cut up the grapefruit pulp and boil for 10 minutes in 8 ounces of distilled water. Strain and combine with the juice from the refrigerator. Sip slowly to bring down fever. For intermittent fevers or flu use six grapefruits and 48 ounces distilled water. Sip slowly throughout the day. Do not eat or drink anything else except water. Continue for 2-3 days or as long as necessary.

To treat fevers of influenza, use 2 teaspoons peach tree leaves in 1 cup boiling water. Cool, strain, and take 1 tablespoon every hour.

Combine 1 ounce feverweed and 1 pint boiling water to make a tea. Drink this tea freely instead of water to bring down fevers.

The fresh bark of button bush is good for recurring fever. Make a tea using ½ teaspoon root or bark and 1 cup boiling water. Add one teaspoon honey and boil until the mixture is syrupy. Take 1 teaspoon every hour.

For fever and fatigue, combine 5-20 grains cayenne with 1 quart boiling water for 10 minutes. Add 1 teaspoon honey and 1 cup orange juice. This treatment will help reduce fever and restore equilibrium. Sip slowly.

Pneumonia

Warm ½ cup of goosegrease and have the patient drink it. Give lemon to help get rid of the taste. Place a hot water bottle at the feet and cover the patient well. During the night, the patient will sweat heavily. Witnesses of this treatment say that the pneumonia will be gone in the morning.

Giant solomon seal is a good treatment for chest infections. Take in a tea and make into a poultice. Use only the root. For tea use 1 teaspoon solomon seal to 1 cup boiling water and drink three cups per day. Change the poultice when dry and reapply.

To control bleeding of the lungs, mix 2 ounces slippery elm bark with 1 quart warm milk. Take 1 teaspoon every ½ hour to soothe the membranes of the lungs.

Rub oil of cloves into the chest to treat all chest ailments. This will help to break tension and clear breathing passages. Give 1 drop oil of cloves with 1 teaspoon honey once or twice a day. This treatment is also effective for tuberculosis.

DIGESTIVE SYSTEM

Each organ of the digestive system, the mouth, throat, stomach, intestines and rectum, is dependent upon the preceeding organ to have done their job properly. A malfunction in one organ will drastically affect the functioning of the others.

The Mouth
The mouth is the first organ of the digestive system. If you chew properly, the food you swallow will already be partially digested and the body will already have begun to assimilate the vitamins and minerals contained in the food.

For water brash (burping foods or liquids into the mouth) chew a small piece of calamus slowly and swallow the juice to help bring relief. Children should be given a weak tea made with ½ teaspoon of calamus to 1 cup boiling water. Give only cooled tea to children.

Arsesmart herb is an excellent gargle for thrush (mouth ulcers) and sore throats. Use 1 ounce leaves in 1 pint cold water. Drink 3 ounces when thirsty in place of water, or gargle 3-5 times per day. This tea is an antibiotic that has no side effects.

Charcoal sweetens the breath and aids the digestive system by absorbing odors and gas.

For halitosis, mix 1 teaspoon aromatized sodium perborate with ½ glass warm water. Rinse out the mouth in the morning and evening, do not swallow.

Chlorophyl, found in all green plants, helps absorb breath odors. Eat fresh parseley, watercress, or chickweed when needed.

The Throat

Sage tea is an excellent gargle for sore throats. Use 1 teaspoon sage to 1 cup boiling water. Steep several minutes and strain. Gargle and sip morning and evening as needed.

Gargle with pure (or diluted) lemon juice one hour and black tea the next hour alternately to relieve sore throat and laryngitis. Do not drink the black non-herbal tea, but the tannic acid it contains is good for soothing the throat when used as directed with the lemon.

Aids to Digestion

The body manufactures certain enzymes which break down starches and modify proteins to prepare them for use by the body. Some of these enzymes are found in brewer's yeast, raw honey, pollen, rosehips and kelp. Papayas are particularly high in protein modifying enzymes. Eating adequate amounts of these foods will boost production of digestive enzymes.

Plaintain soothes and tones the internal organs. Use 1 teaspoon herb to 1 cup boiling water and drink two cups per day for 3-4 days.

Mix bileberry with equal parts thyme, strawberry leaves, and hyssop. Use 1 teaspoon herbs mixed with 1 cup boiling water and drink cold. This tea soothes the bowels and helps increase the body's resistance to disease.

Agrimony is good for all digestive disorders. Use in capsule or powder form and take 5 grains three times a day.

Burdock is good for all digestive disorders. Use 1 teaspoon to 1 cup boiling water and steep for 10 minutes. Drink 3 cups per day.

Cinnamon helps tone the bowels. Use ¼ teaspoon in 1 cup boiling water. Take 1 cup per day.

Colic

Colic is caused by gas in the system. The child may have gotten this from the mother, or when formula is used, it indicates that the mixture is too rich for the child's system. Soy milk formulas can cause colic also, if the mixture needs more dilution.

Horsebain herb helps to relieve colic. Use 1 teaspoon of the powdered leaves to 1 cup boiling water. Give ½-1 cup cooled mixture when needed.

☆Camomile tea is a good treatment for colic. Use ¼ teaspoon camomile flowers to 1 cup boiling water and steep for 5-10 minutes. Sweeten with honey and give warm. Test for temperature.

Lovage tea helps ease the pain of colic. Use ¼ teaspoon herb to 1 cup boiling water and steep for 3 minutes. Give ½ cup of cooled mixture. Sweeten with honey if desired.

Gas and Heartburn

Gas is created when the food is not properly chewed and by drinking with meals, as this process lessens the effectiveness of the salivary glands and impedes digestion. Eat slowly without liquids and relax while dining.

Gas may also be created by improper cooking. Beans contain many toxins which create gas if not properly cooked. To reduce the toxins and add to your enjoyment, here is a recipe for cooking beans.

Soak dried beans overnight and in the morning pour off the water. Add fresh water and 1 onion and bring to a boil. Strain off the water and throw out the onion. This wash will absorb the toxins in the beans which create gas. Replenish the water and add spices and herbs to taste. Cook until the beans are soft and well done. Eat only in small quantities as the body does not need excessive amounts of protein.

Ginger, taken after a heavy meal, is an aid to digestion and helps prevent flatulance. Use ¼ teaspoon to 1 cup hot water, steep 5 minutes and sip slowly.

Angelica is a valuable treatment for digestive trouble. Use 2 ounces angelica, ¼ ounce fennel, ¼ ounce anise, and 1 ounce coriander. Grind into a powder and mix with 8 ounces pure alcohol. Let mixture stand for eight days, then add 1 pound honey mixed with 2½ pints tepid water. Take 1 tablespoon morning and evening to relieve gas.

Catnip tea, taken warm, is helpful for gas. Use 1 pinch tea to ½ cup boiling water. Steep five minutes and then sip slowly when needed.

Fresh cleaver's herb, when cooked with beans, adds flavor and minimizes production of gas.

Parsley is an efficient treatment for gas. Eat fresh and raw or make into a tea using 1 teaspoon parsley to 1 cup boiling water.

Eat orange peels a few minutes after the meal to aid digestion.

Bay leaves make a pleasant tea which helps tone and strengthen the digestive organs and helps expel gas from both the stomach and the bowels. Use ½ teaspoon bay leaves to 1 cup boiling water. Sip slowly.

Slippery elm bark neutralizes stomach acid and helps to absorb gases. It contains enzymes which help digestion. Make a tea using 1 teaspoon slippery elm bark or powder to 1 cup boiling water. Sip slowly.

Combine ½ teaspoon wild clover, 1 teaspoon lemon juice and 1 cup boiling water. Take 1 tablespoon of the tea 3-5 times a day for gas.

For indigestion, mix ground horseradish with as much cream as it will absorb and eat slowly.

Camomile tea helps soothe intestinal disorders, gas and cramps. Use 1 teaspoon herb to 1 cup boiling water and drink several cups per day.

☆Peppermint tea aids the digestive processes, when taken one hour after a meal. Make a tea using 1 teaspoon peppermint leaves to 1 cup boiling water and sip slowly.

Make a tea using ½ teaspoon each of cardamon seed and meadowsweet or horehound herb with 1 cup boiling water. Steep 3-5 minutes and sip slowly for heartburn.

Dill weed contains oils which relax the stomach. Use 1 teaspoon seeds in 1 cup water, boil for 15 minutes, strain and drink slowly. This tea will help absorb gas and stop hiccups.

Combine 1 ounce gentian root, ½ ounce colombo root, and ½ ounce skullcap and cover with two pints cold water. Simmer slowly for 20 minutes and drink 1 hour before and 2 hours after meals. This is an effective, gentle treatment for elderly people suffering from indigestion.

Unground mustard seeds are an excellent treatment for gastritis. Take 1 seed the first day, 2 the second day, 3 the third day, adding one seed per day until 20 seeds are being taken. Then reduce the number by one seed each day until back down to 1. Swallow the seeds with water first thing in the morning on an empty stomach.

Allspice helps relieve gas from the upper intestinal tract. Use ½ teaspoon to 1 cup boiling water and drink one cup per day or chew ¼ teaspoon allspice and swallow.

Simple indigestion and heartburn can be relieved by sipping the juice of one-half of a fresh lemon in 1 cup tepid water with 1 teaspoon soda. Drink the mixture immediately.

The Stomach

Blood root helps to stimulate the gastric and intestinal secretions and aids digestion. Use 1/12 grain of bloodroot to 1 cup boiling water and sip slowly. Take two cups per day.

Buck bean root is good for improving digestion. Make a tea using 1 teaspoon root to 1 cup boiling water. Slowly swallow a large mouthful three times a day. This tea is bitter but effective.

Use 1 ounce prickly ash in 1 pint boiling water to make a stomach tonic. Steep the mixture 15 minutes and drink 3-4 cups per day.

Lovage is useful for all disorders of the stomach and urinary tract. Use 1 teaspoon herb to 1 cup boiling water and drink 4 cups per day.

Ground ivy is a good treatment for lead colic. Use 1 teaspoon ivy to 1 cup boiling water and drink 2 cups per day.

Garlic will help to relieve gas, heartburn, stomach upset, and all forms of indigestion as it destroys dangerous organisms in the system without harming the necessary bacteria.

Stomach Cramps

☆Parseley tea will help to relieve stomach cramps. Make a tea using 1 teaspoon fresh or dried parseley to 1 cup boiling water. Steep 4-5 minutes and sip slowly.

To help soothe stomach cramps, make a tea using 1 teaspoon valarian root or leaves to 1 cup boiling water. Drink 2-3 cups per day.

St. John's wort helps soothe stomach pain. Use ½ teaspoon wort to 1 cup boiling water and drink 1 cup three times a day.

Stomach Ulcers

Ulcers are usually caused by tension. If you will reorganize your life to eliminate heavy pressures and stress, many ulcers will disappear. Vitamins A, C, and E will soothe stomach ulcers. It is always more beneficial to get the vitamins you need from the food you eat rather than supplements. See the appendices for lists of foods which are high in these vitamins.

Stomach disorders will respond to raw juices, particularly carrot, celery, cabbage, tomato and parseley juice. Use few or no spices. Vitamin E should be added to the diet to help clear up all stomach conditions.

Cucumber juice is good for stomach and bladder ulcers. Drink several cups a day.

A strict diet of avocadoes will help to heal ulcers. For two weeks, eat nothing but avocadoes and sip at least 3 glasses of water per day.

Carrot juice is nourishing and soothing for stomach ulcers. Drink ½ cup three times a day.

Parseley juice and alfalfa promote healing of ulcers. Drink 1 cup parseley juice morning and evening or take 1 tablespoon parseley 3-4 times a day. Alfalfa tablets may be taken morning and evening after meals.

Papayas contain enzymes which replenish the stomach lining and help with protein digestion. Make a tea using ½ teaspoon powder or root to 1 cup boiling water. Steep several minutes and drink one cup per day. This tea is particularly beneficial if you eat large quantities of meat.

Balm helps to relieve chronic stomach conditions including ulcers. Make a tea using ½ teaspoon balm to 1 pint boiling water. Steep several minutes, strain, and drink 3 cups per day.

Mix gentian, wormwood, comdurango and American century in equal parts. Use 1 teaspoon of the mixture to 1 cup boiling water and steep for 3-5 minutes. Drink 2 cups per day for ulcers.

Green elder bark tea will promote healing of ulcers. Use 1 teaspoon bark to 1 cup boiling water and steep for 5 minutes. Strain and drink three cups per day.

Barley helps to rebuild the lining of the stomach and soothes stomach ulcers because it contains vitamins B_1 and B_2.

For ulcers, take ½ teaspoon powdered cloves or ½ teaspoon oil of cloves. Hold in the mouth until dissolved and mixed well with the saliva. Repeat this treatment three times a day.

Take 1 teaspoon concentrated licorice syrup daily and eat foods high in B_{12} (see appendices for sources.) Continue treatment daily for ulcers.

Comfrey and pepsin are recommended for ulcerative colitis. They will help soothe the digestive tract and dissolve mucous from the walls of the intestines. Make a tea with 1 teaspoon mixed comfrey and pepsin to 1 cup boiling water and set aside. Boil 3 tablespoons flaxseed in 1 pint of water for 5 minutes and strain. Add the comfrey-pepsin tea and drink at once.

Persimmons are a high energy food and will promote healing of ulcers by soothing the mucous membranes in the digestive tract. Eat 1 persimmon a day.

The following diet is recommended for treatment of peptic ulcers:
On day one, eat nothing and drink 1 pint fresh carrot juice.
On day two, eat nothing, drink 10 ounces carrot juice, 3 ounces spinach juice and 2 ounces parseley juice.
On day three, eat nothing, drink 1 pint each of spinach juice, celery juice and carrot juice.

Constipation
Proper elimination is absolutely necessary for good health. When nutritive supplies are insufficient, the body lacks the energy needed to evacuate the bowels as completely and frequently as necessary. If your body is in good condition, and you are eating the proper foods, you should have three bowel movements per day. Foods which are high in vitamins A, B, C, E, G and K will help to relieve constipation. These vitamins are found in large quantities in cashews, Jerusalem artichokes, spinach, prunes, persimmons, mangoes, bell peppers, cranberries and cranberry juice, cucumbers, asparagus, green beans, bamboo shoots, and all roughage foods such as bean sprouts and lettuce.

A pantothenic acid deficiency can cause constipation and other digestive disorders. Pantothenic acid is found in royal jelly, honey, human milk, peanuts, broccoli and most other vegetables.

Laxatives

Yerba mate stimulates peristalsis and nourishes the intestinal tract. It is a high source of vitamin C. Take 1 teaspoon yerba mate to 1 cup boiling water and drink several cups per day.

☆Dandelion is useful for all types of constipation and will help strengthen the stomach. Use fresh in salads or make a tea using 1 teaspoon of the root to 1 cup boiling water. Steep for ½ hour, and drink 1-2 cups daily.

Cascara bark helps tone the bowels and aids elimination. Take 1 tablespoon before bedtime in tablet or capsule form. Do not exceed dosage.

Wormwood is an excellent, fast-acting laxative. Use ½ teaspoon wormwood to 1 cup boiling water and sip slowly. Do not drink more than 1 cup in a 24 hour period.

Black root is good for constipation. Use 1-2 teaspoons per cup of boiling water. Steep for 10 minutes. Black root helps remove obstructions of the digestive tract.

Pumpkin seeds are excellent for constipation. Chew one teaspoon of seeds per day. Pumpkin seeds are high in male hormones and are not recommended for women.

American senna is an effective laxative. Use 1 teaspoon leaves or 5 pods to 1 cup boiling water, let steep ½ hour, and drink ½ cup morning and evening.

Masterwort herb stimulates the digestive organs and absorbs gases from the intestines. Use ½ teaspoon to 1 cup boiling water. Drink 1 cup per day.

Black elder bark is a good laxative. Use 1 teaspoon bark to 1 cup boiling water. Take 1 cup per day.

American bearsfoot root stimulates the glands, relieves pain and is an effective laxative. Use 1 teaspoon to 1 cup boiling water and take at bedtime.

Soak fresh cucumbers in kelp water overnight and drink in the morning before breakfast. This mixture relieves congestion which causes nausea and is an excellent laxative.

A lack of B vitamins will cause constipation. Eat 1 yeast cake per day for several months to tone the bowels and relieve constipation. Comfrey tea, papaya and chlorophyll tablets are also helpful.

The inner bark of the white ash tree is a useful treatment for constipation. Steep a heaping teaspoon in 1 cup boiling water for 30 minutes and drink ½ glass in the morning and in the evening.

Use 1 teaspoon each of buckhorn bark, indian senna pods and bladderwrack in two cups boiling water. Steep 10 minutes, strain and take ½ cup morning and evening for two days for constipation.

Eating 2-3 fresh tomatoes daily before breakfast helps to keep the bowels regular.

May apples will soothe the bowels and relieve constipation. Use 1 teaspoon may apple leaves to 1 pint boiling water and take 1 teaspoon per day.

Bamboo shoots may be used for constipation and intestinal poisoning. Eat raw or cover with boiling water for 10 minutes to soften. Eat about ½ cup per day.

Soak 1 tablespoon whole flaxseed and 1 tablespoon wheat bran in 1 cup vegetable broth overnight. In the morning heat, blend well, and drink. Do not strain or chew. This mixture will help to restore normal peristalsis rhythm. Do not use during a fast.

To soothe the intestines and restore regularity to the bowels eat only tree ripened figs and salads with a dressing made of lemon and apple juice for 1 day each week. Figs help to re-establish the acid-alkaline balance in the system. and ease colitis.

Vervain helps to remove obstructions of the colon. Use 1 teaspoon of the powdered plant to 1 cup boiling water and drink 1 cup every hour until results are obtained.

Persimmons will soothe the digestive tract and help relieve constipation, colitis, and sore throats.

In an emergency, olive oil will help to relieve constipation. Sip small amounts (up to 1 cup) throughout the day until results are obtained. Lemon juice may be taken to cut the oily taste.

Diarrhea

Diarrhea is a symptom and not a disease. It indicates that the body is ridding itself of intruding organisms or excessive wastes from overeating.

Garlic will destroy harmful bacteria, but will not destroy beneficial bacteria found in the intestinal tract. Use in tea or eat raw in salads.

Cold raspberry leaf tea is an excellent treatment for diarrhea. Use 1 ounce leaves to ½ pint water, simmer together for 20 minutes. Drink cold. Use ½ ounce herb to ½ pint water to treat diarrhea in babies.

Use 1 teaspoon ginger root to 1 cup boiling water and take 3 cups per day for diarrhea.

Apricots help to check diarrhea. Eat 3 whole apricots per day.

Swamp dogwood is a good treatment for diarrhea and dyspepsia. Make into a tea using 1 teaspoon swamp dogwood leaves or bark in 1 cup boiling water. Drink 3 cups per day.

Use 1 ounce powdered slippery elm in 1 quart boiling water and simmer down to 1 pint. Take 1 teaspoon every ½ hour to soothe the membranes of the intestinal tract. Honey may be added if needed. For infants or elderly people, cover slippery elm powder with milk and eat like cereal.

Peruvian rhatany is a useful treatment for diarrhea to restore normal functioning of the bowels. Use ½ teaspoon powdered root to 1 cup boiling water and take 2 cups per day.

Blueberries and huckleberries will help to relieve discomfort of diarrhea. Eat 5-20 fresh berries or bake in a pie made with honey.

Mix equal parts bileberry leaves, thyme and strawberry with 1 cup boiling water and drink cold to help control diarrhea. Honey may be added if necessary.

Make a tea using 1 teaspoon black elder bark or leaves and 1 cup boiling water. Sweeten with honey and take 1 cup per day to help diarrhea.

Dysentery can be treated with 2 tablespoons epsom salts and 1 glass water. Drink quickly.

Boil whole Canada thistles in milk to make a soothing remedy for dysentery.

Juniper berries are helpful in the treatment of dysentery. Use 5 berries to 1 cup boiling water and drink ½ cup twice a day.

Barley is a body builder and will help to control diarrhea as it contains vitamins B_1 and B_2. Use in cereals, soups and stews.

Hemorrhoids and Piles

Hemorrhoids may be caused by pressure on the rectum from unassimilated bulk foods, often this pressure increases during pregnancy. But overeating is the most common cause. When you have eaten too much food, the body is unable to digest it properly and the fecal matter will remain hard and lumpy and strain the muscles and veins of the anus.

To relieve pain of hemorrhoids, apply a poultice of cottage cheese to the anus. Change poultice three times per day until relief is obtained.

Juniper berries are useful for treatment of hemorrhoids. Put 4-5 berries in 1 pint boiling water and steep for ½ hour. Drink 4 cups per day.

Pilewort is a useful treatment for hemorrhoids and will help draw the tissues together. Use 1 ounce herb to 1 pint boiling water and take ½ cup twice a day.

Blue flag juice eases pain of piles and hemorrhoids. Use 10-20 drops in ½ cup water or 1 ounce powder to 1 pint water. Drink ½ cup three times per day.

Steep black elder flowers in olive oil for two weeks and rub onto the skin outside the anus to relieve pain of hemorrhoids.

Mullein flowers will help relieve hemorrhoid pain. Use 1 ounce powdered leaves in 1 pint milk. Boil for 10 minutes and strain, drink 3 cups per day.

A clove of garlic placed in the rectum helps reduce swelling of hemorrhoids.

☆Use fresh comfrey leaves in a poultice to draw tissues of hemorrhoids back into place and help relieve the pain. If you do not have fresh comfrey, use the dried root or leaves. Make a strong tea by pouring boiling water over the herb. Use the softened roots and leaves in the poultice and drink the comfrey tea. This procedure will help to clear hemorrhoids completely.

Soak a piece of cotton with papaya juice and place against the rectum to draw out the irritation and stop the bleeding of piles and hemorrhoids.

Soften sicklewort leaves with boiling water and make into a poultice. Place the poultice against the rectum to help stop bleeding of piles.

EARS

The ears are vital sensory organs and need adequate supplies of vitamins A and C. These vitamins are beneficial for ear infections, pain or deafness. High sources of A and C are carrots, carrot juice, parseley and all citrus fruits. See the appendices for further information.

Ear Noise

Ringing in the ears can be treated with summer savory. Use ½ teaspoon herb to ½ cup boiling water and steep for several minutes. Mix 1 teaspoon of this mixture with 1 teaspoon oil of roses. When cool, place one drop of the mixture in each ear to help ease the ringing sensation. Repeat once a week until hearing clears. In addition, massage the neck behind and in front of each ear then pull gently as directed by the numbers and arrows in diagram 4. Repeat daily.

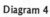

Diagram 4

Ear Discharge

Combine equal quantities of black currant leaves, honeysuckle, horehound and giant hyssop. Use 1 teaspoon of this mixture to 1 cup boiling water. Put 1 drop of the warm liquid in each ear. DO NOT USE HOT. Repeat once a week to help clear discharge.

☆Earaches and Infections

Ear infections may be treated by boiling 1 clove of garlic in ½ cup water until soft but not mushy. Lay cooled clove on the outside of the ear, but do not push down ear canal! Cover with a piece of clean cotton and hold in place with scotch tape. Leave poultice for several days (changing daily) until infection is drawn out.

Make a strong tea of mullein flowers using 1 teaspoon to ½ cup boiling water. Mix 1 tablespoon of this mixture with 1 tablespoon olive oil and let stand overnight. Use 1 drop of this liquid in each ear two times a week to help ease the ache.

Devil's walking stick seeds, when crushed, yield an oil which aids earache pain. Use 1 drop in affected ear once a week.

One pinch of dried yarrow leaves and 1 tablespoon boiling water mixed together and steeped for 5 minutes helps both earaches and infections. Use 1 drop in each ear once a week until condition clears.

One drop garlic oil in each ear helps clear ear infections. Use warm, not hot, oil and repeat once a week.

Ear Mites

One drop of warmed camphor-phenique in each ear is a good treatment for ear mites. After one week use a small amount (3-5 drops) hydrogen peroxide in affected ear and allow to drain. The mites will come out with the liquid.

Deafness

Raw garlic and onion juice taken internally once a day can help to restore hearing. Use about two ounces of the combined mixture daily.

Summer savory is excellent for deafness. Use 1 ounce of the herb to 1 pint boiling water, steep several minutes and strain. Drink 3 cups daily.

Mullein flowers steeped in olive oil for 2 weeks will make a good ointment for deafness. Use 1 drop in each ear once a week and massage the outside of the ear, both back and front, daily.

Angelica juice dropped into the ear is helpful in deafness. Put one drop in each ear once a week.

Ear Wax
To soften ear wax deposits in the ears, press firmly but gently behind the ear, in front of the ear, and then pull the ear lobe up and down. (See diagram 4) This procedure also stimulates ear circulation and should be repeated daily.

EYES

The eyes are sensory organs and, as such, they need plenty of vitamin C. Deficiencies in any of the vitamins or minerals will show up first in the eyes as little "bloodshot" lines corresponding to the area of the body which is malfunctioning. Irisdiagnosis, while not included here, is becoming more widely practiced as a method of early detection and prevention of disease.

To Improve Vision
Mix the following ingredients in a blender and drink slowly before meals. Continue for two weeks to help improve vision.
- ¼ cup grapefruit juice
- ¼ cup apple juice
- ¼ cup orange juice
- 2 tablespoons wheat germ oil
- 1 tablespoon unfiltered honey
- 2 tablespoons apple cider vinegar

Pour 1 quart boiling water over 1 cup fresh parsley to make a tonic for the eyes. Steep for 15 minutes, strain, and drink 3 cups per day. Keep this tonic refrigerated.

Calcium and vitamin D are helpful for both near and far-sightedness. See the appendices for foods which contain these vitamins and use daily.

Three teaspoons of sunflower seeds per day contain high amounts of vitamins necessary to help vision.

Vitamin E helps clear foggy vision. Start taking small doses and build up slowly over several weeks to 400-800 i.u. daily.

To help strengthen the eyes, just before bedtime place a lighted candle even with the top of the head and sit 1½ feet away. Sit erect, with the feet together. Hold the eyelids open with the index fingers and look at the candle without blinking for 5 minutes. Don't wipe away the tears as wiping may bruise the eyes. Repeat this procedure for five minutes every other night for two weeks. Stop for two weeks and then begin again. Continue until vision is strengthened.

To improve the eyes place the index fingers at the outside corners of the eyes and do not press. Squeeze the eyes and relax several times. This helps to build the muscles of the eyes. See diagram 5.

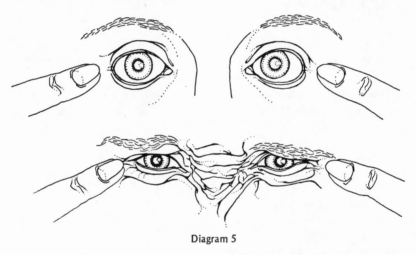

Diagram 5

To improve the eyes use maidenhair and green ginger, ½ teaspoon of each with ½ cup boiling water. Put 1 drop in each eye morning and evening until the eye film has cleared.

Rosemary tea helps to strengthen sight. Use 1 teaspoon rosemary to 1 cup boiling water and put 1 drop in each eye morning and evening. Drink the rest of the cup of tea.

☆Sage tea helps keep the eyes bright and also improves the memory. Use 1 teaspoon sage to 1 cup boiling water and drink freely throughout the day. One cup daily for six months helps to clear and cleanse the eyes.

Tea made with juniper berries helps to strengthen sight. Use several berries to 1 cup boiling water. Drink 3 cups per day.

Rutin strengthens the eyes by helping to decrease capillary tension. Take 1 tablet four times during the day (about 400mg.)

Sore and Inflamed Eyes

Violet leaves, in tea and a poultice, help bring down swelling and draw out soreness from the eyes. Use 1 teaspoon leaves to 1 cup boiling water. Steep for 5 minutes, strain and use strained leaves in a poultice on the eyes for 15 minutes. Drink the liquid.

Use grated or scraped raw Irish potatoes in a poultice on the eyes. This helps to relieve swelling or soreness. Use poultice nightly for 15 minutes. This procedure may be repeated in the morning if needed.

Adder's tongue herb made into a tea with horsetail herb is good for sore eyes. Use ½ teaspoon each in 1 cup boiling water. Steep for 5 minutes and strain. Sip slowly two cups per day.

For sore eyes make an eye wash with the following ingredients. Combine herbs with water and steep for 20 minutes. Cool and wash eyes with the mixture each morning and evening until soreness is gone.
    ½ teaspoon fit root
    ½ teaspoon fennel seed
    1 pint boiling water

Swollen eyes can be soothed by making a poultice of grated apple and laying it over the eyes for 15-20 minutes. This will help draw out the swelling and relieve the irritation. Fresh corn silk, papaya or witch hazel poultices may be used instead of apple.

☆Lemon juice is a cleansing eyewash, especially when you have been exposed to dust, long hours under harsh lights or work with printing compounds. This is a good all round eyewash which will clean and soothe the eyes and help restore normal functioning. Use 1 drop lemon juice (fresh only!) in 1 eyecup (or 1 ounce) warm water and wash each eye. Never rub the eyes.

Pursaline herb, used in a poultice, helps relieve inflammations. Bruise the herb before placing it in the cloth and lay over the eyes for 15-20 minutes.

A poultice of bruised ivy, placed on the eyelids for 15 minutes, helps relieve swelling.

Bags Under the Eyes

☆ Bags under the eyes can be caused by water retention, stress, or most commonly, loss of sleep. Make a poultice by using black tea (orange pekoe, etc.) bags, moistened and laid over the eyes. This will help to draw out the dark circles. Grated potato, apple, papaya leaves, cucumber or alfalfa will also draw out circles and relax tension behind the eyes.

Eye Infections

Mix together one teaspoon canned evaporated milk and 1 drop spirit of camphor. Put 1 drop mixture in each eye morning and evening to help clear eye infections.

Two drops pure flaxseed oil in each eye morning and evening will help clear eye infections.

Conjunctivitis can be cleared by eating goat milk yogurt and using yogurt in a poultice on the eyes daily. It helps to destroy the bacteria in the system which causes the infection.

"Pink eye" can be cleared almost overnight by using grated apple in a poultice placed over the eyes. Leave on for 20 minutes. Repeat daily if needed.

For eye infections, use a tea made with dried quince seeds. Use ¼ teaspoon seeds in ½ cup boiling water. Steep until cool, then put 1 drop in each eye morning and evening for 1 week to clear up infection.

One clary seed, placed into the eye, will help to work out foreign objects in the eye. It will work around the eye to draw out the object. The seeds, made into a tea, will help strengthen the eyes and remove film from the eyes. Use 1 teaspoon seeds to 1 cup boiling water and allow tea to stand overnight before drinking.

Calcium helps to cleanse the eyes when the pigment layers are inflamed. Make a solution with 2 mg. calcium dissolved in ½ cup warm water. Wash the eyes with this liquid morning and evening for 1 week. Use warm solution each time.

Chapped Eyelids
For chapped eyelids gently rub the eyelids with witch hazel on a cotton ball. Repeat 2-3 times per day.

To Cleanse Babies' Eyes
Mix together dried poppy flower and lavender flowers in equal quantities. Use ½ teaspoon mixture to 1 cup boiling water, steep 5 minutes and strain. When mixture is cool use to cleanse eyes morning and evening as needed.

Black Eyes
To reduce swelling and bruises of black eyes, use equal parts lard and salt in a poultice and place over the eyes. This stimulates the circulation which helps the body eliminate dead and bruised cells.

Tired Eyes
To soothe tired eyes, use a pad of cotton dampened with witch hazel or rosemary tea and placed over the eyelids for 10-15 minutes. Grated apples in a poultice are also effective.

Red Eyes
Grapevine juice, used a tiny drop in each eye, will help reddened eyes. The juice will sting but will help to clear the eyes quickly.

Dimming of Sight
Slit open white willow bark or crush the leaves and collect the liquid. One drop of the sap morning and evening in each eye will reduce redness of the eyes and improve dimming eyesight. This treatment is also helpful for removing film over the eyes. Repeat daily until condition clears.

Cover dragon flowers with distilled water and let stand overnight. Use 1 drop of the liquid in each eye morning and evening to improve eyesight.

One clary seed, dropped into the eye, will float around inside the eye and clean infection and help remove film. The seed will work itself out when the cleansing is completed. Repeat this procedure several times a day for severe infections. Follow this treatment with 3-4 drops of pure, fresh cream in the eye to ease the inflammation of the mucous membranes.

Spots Before the Eyes

Spots before the eyes indicate congestion in the system. If the spots are black they indicate congestion in the liver. Drink sesame seed tea using 1 teaspoon seeds to 1 cup boiling water, steep 5-10 minutes, strain and drink 2-3 cups per day. If the spots are white flecks, they indicate that the kidneys are not getting enough water to flush out the toxins. Be sure you are sipping, not gulping at least 3 eight ounce glasses of water a day. See the liver section for more information about cleansing congestion.

Night Blindness

Watercress contains many vitamins and minerals which help restore night vision. Eat daily in salads or make into a tea using fresh herb.

Carrots and carrot juice help restore night vision. Eat 2-3 carrots per day or drink 4 ounces carrot juice.

Bloodshot Eyes

Bloodshot eyes, except when caused by wind exposure, usually indicate a need for more vitamin B in the system. Eat sprouted grains, sunflower seeds and other foods high in B-complex vitamins daily.

Sunburned Eyes

For sunburned eyes, use grated apple in a poultice and drink lemon juice and water combined.

Stys

When stys occur eat no eggs, fish, or chicken. Collect your urine from the first elimination in the morning and dab onto the sty.

☆Cysts on the Eyes

The white inner lining of the orange skin contains vitamins F and P which help dissolve eye cysts. Take 6 tablespoons hourly for one day and make a tea using 1 teaspoon orange skin to 1 cup boiling water to use as eye drops. Put 1 drop of the tea in the affected eye one or two times per day. This substance also helps reduce swelling. Use only organic oranges and continue until condition clears.

Cysts on the eye can be treated with 1 drop of your own urine from the first elimination of the morning. This treatment can also be used for blurred vision.

Alfalfa is excellent for treating blurred vision and other conditions of the eyes. Dissolve one tablet in 1 cup boiling water and put 1 drop cooled liquid in each eye daily.

Cataracts and Glaucoma

Cataracts indicate a deficiency of B vitamins, especially B_2 (riboflavin.) One heaping teaspoon daily of this vitamin is an effective treatment. Glaucoma and cataracts also indicate the need for vitamins A, C, E, rutin and calcium. A healthy diet, including foods which contain these vitamins, plus daily supplements will help to alleviate this condition.

Caladine greater has been used in the treatment of cataracts for hundreds of years. Press the leaves and collect the liquid which should be dropped into the eye 2 times a day. Operations can often be avoided with this treatment.

☆Place the yellow side of a piece of organic orange peel over the eye and leave overnight. On the second night, use the white side of a fresh piece of organic orange peel. If the peel over the eye creates a great deal of heat, remove it and try again the next night. Continue each night alternating the side of the peel until condition is cleared. Use fresh peel each night and use only organic oranges as commercial oranges have been sprayed with chemicals.

For treatment of glaucoma, take daily supplements of vitamins A, C, B, E, and calcium and apply golden seal tincture to the cornea in a solution of 2 drops in 1 ounce warm water three times per day. This treatment is also good for ulcers of the cornea.

Glaucoma sufferers should not drink coffee as caffeine is hard on the blood vessels of the eyes. Dandelion coffee, which is made from the dried root of dandelion, may be substituted.

Rosehips are an excellent treatment for glaucoma and cataracts. Make a tea using 1 teaspoon rosehips to 1 cup boiling water and drink at least three or more cups per day.

FEET AND LEGS

The feet are, without question, the most abused part of the body. They are constantly under stress and pressure from tight shoes, heat and cold, and from all physical activity. Corns, calluses and blisters on the feet should call attention to abuse, but even tired feet affect every organ in the body. Here are some ways of pepping up not only your feet—but the entire system. Foot massages stimulate every organ in the body, relieve tension, and help to regulate the digestion. The foot massage charts (diagrams 6 and 7) show where nerve endings for the various organs are located in the feet. All diseases may be treated by massaging the corresponding area of the foot.

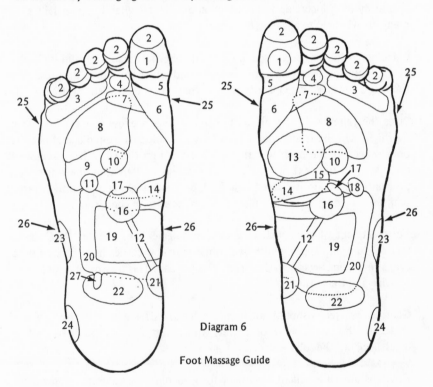

Diagram 6

Foot Massage Guide

1. pituitary gland 2. sinuses and top of head. 3. ears 4. eyes 5. neck 6. thyroid
7. bronchial tubes 8. lungs 9. liver 10. solar plexus|11. gall bladder 12. kidney tubes
13. heart 14. pancreas 15. stomach 16. kidney 17.adrenal glands 18. spleen
19. small intestine 20. large intestine 21. bladder 22. sex glands and organs 23. hip
24. knee 25. shoulder line 26. waist line 27. appendix.

1. glands

2. kidneys

3. shoulder and neck tension

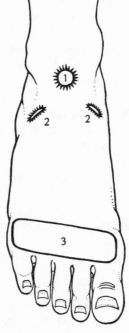

Diagram 7

Tired Feet
Mix two tablespoons each of camomile, peppermint, oatstraw, red clover, elderberry leaves, linden flowers, fennel, dock, rosehips and alfalfa in 1 quart
cold water. Bring to a boil and simmer for 15 minutes, cool and soak the feet
for 10-15 minutes in the liquid.

Hot, Itchy Feet
Soak the feet for 15 minutes in warm water from boiled potatoes. Dry feet in
a towel with sea salt or dulse powder sprinkled in it, then massage the feet
with 2 tablespoons sesame or almond oil.

Cold Feet
Cold feet are usually caused by nervousness which inhibits the circulation. A
small amount of cayenne pepper sprinkled into the shoes helps to stimulate
the circulation and correct the condition.

Cramps in the Legs and Feet
B-complex vitamins, taken daily, help to ease toe cramps.

Leg and foot cramps indicate an improper assimilation of calcium in the system caused by a lack of vitamins D and E. Sipping a glass of warm water and lemon juice nightly helps supply these vitamins.

Raspberry leaves, taken in tea, help soothe cramping muscles and are nutritionally beneficial. Use 1 teaspoon leaves to one cup boiling water and steep 5 minutes. Sip slowly, 2-3 cups per day as needed.

The treatments listed before are helpful for tired muscles in any part of the body.

To massage the legs, elevate the feet and legs and slap the legs as hard as possible with open palms.

Fallen Arches
Mix 1 ounce powdered wormwood and 1 pint pure alcohol (or rum) and allow mixture to stand for one week. Shake the bottle each night. Strain and rub on the feet morning and evening and bind the feet with gauze. Continue for 3-4 weeks and take supplements of calcium and vitamin D.

Foot Odor
Wash the feet with green soap and soak them in apple cider vinegar water for 10 minutes. Soak the socks in a separate batch of solution and then dry. Repeat daily. Check the diet to be sure sufficient zinc is being supplied.

Puncture Wounds in the Feet
☆Puncture wounds from rusty nails and unclean objects, should be sterilized and the toxins drawn out with a poultice of pouch tobacco. Mix the tobacco with enough water to make a paste. This poultice will help to draw out the poisons and reduce swelling and soreness. Use the poultice at least for 24 hours, changing several times or until all swelling and soreness is gone. This treatment will help prevent lockjaw and tetanus.

Ingrown Toenails
Ingrown toenails may be caused by wearing shoes which are too tight or by

cutting the nails incorrectly. The shoe size should be changed immediately as the nerve endings for various organs in the body may be affected as well as the foot. The toenails should be trimmed straight across and not rounded at the corners to prevent ingrown toenails.

Mix alum with a little water to make a paste and place in a poultice on the ingrown toenail. This will help to draw out the pain and clear the condition. An alum poultice may be used for any type of foot infection.

To prevent ingrown toenails, scratch the top of the nail with an emory board until the toenail is thin. Repeat daily and the nail will grow out flat.

Varicose Veins
Varicose veins are caused by excess cholesterol in the system and may be treated with daily lecithin supplements which help to break down the cholesterol deposits. Drink plenty of liquids to help the system remain clean. The legs may be massaged nightly with a mixture of witch hazel and white willow bark made into a tea. Other helpful treatments may be found in the section on the heart and circulatory system.

Frostbite
Mullein flowers steeped in oil for several days may be applied to frostbitten extremities to help restore proper circulation.

Your own urine may be applied to frostbitten areas to help facilitate thawing.

Gout
Gout is a form of arthritis which starts in the big toe. The treatments for this condition are given in the Arthritis section.

FEMALE PROBLEMS

Far more than men, women are abused by modern medical philosophies. Thousands of hysterectomies are performed annually and healthy or potentially healthy organs are removed. Even many medical doctors are cringing at the latest trend toward radical mastectomy.

Very little research has gone into finding harmless, natural methods of contraception. Instead, women are taking chemicals manufactured from pregnant mare urine, the consequences of which we will not be certain for years to come. These chemicals alter the hormonal balance, and women are often unaware that these hormones regulate control of all of the body and not just the ovaries and uterus. Astrological, bio-rhythmic, lunar and mental birth control constitute today's limited alternatives, and they, like the chemicals, are not always foolproof. In the coming years, more time and energy will be spent researching alternatives to chemical birth control. But for now, women are advised to use whatever resources are available to them to discover, effective, non-chemical birth control methods.

For All Female Problems

☆Massage the back of the leg behind the ankle to treat all infections or other female problems. Massaging this part of the leg will help to soothe the organs, relax tension, and stimulate proper circulation to the female organs. This area contains nerve endings which correspond to those of the ovaries and female organs. (See diagram 8).

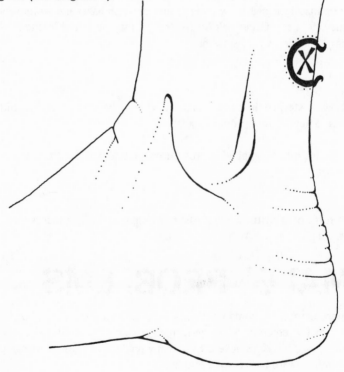

Diagram 8

Vaginal Infections

Vaginal infections indicate that there is an acid-alkaline imbalance in the vagina or uterus. This can result from stress, taking antibiotics, and from birth control methods which change the balance of hormones. A vitamin B deficiency will promote vaginal infections and supplements of this vitamin are recommended for all vaginal infections.

To treat trichomonas and yeast infections, use oatstraw tea to drink, douche with and bathe in. Drink the tea daily for one month to clear up vaginal discharge and strengthen the female organs. Use 1 teaspoon oatstraw to 1 cup boiling water. Make a strong solution of the tea to douche with and do not repeat for at least one week. After douching lie down for at least ½ hour to allow the female organs to return to their proper place. This also allows the tea to completely saturate the uterus before being allowed to leak out. Oatstraw tea may be reused several times before the nutritional benefits are depleted.

☆Vaginal itches and yeast infections respond well to a small poultice of cottage cheese or "farmer's cheese", which is not so wet. Place the poultice on a sanitary napkin and wear daily for two weeks. The cottage cheese will stop the itching and draw the infection out of the system. Change the poultice several times a day depending upon the severity of discharge. This remedy is most effective when oatstraw tea is taken daily. Many women say that eating yogurt restores the bacterial balance in the uterus and helps to stop the discharge.

Red sage helps to stop vaginal discharge. Use 1 pint malt vinegar, 1 ounce powdered red sage and ½ pint cold water. Mix and allow to stand several hours. Take ½ cup several times a day. This mixture works to increase the circulation of the body and strengthen the female organs.

Giant Solomon seal root is helpful in all female ailments. Make a tea using 1 teaspoon root to 1 cup of boiling water or make into a poultice. Drink 2 cups of the tea daily in conjunction with a poultice for best results.

Dandelion is an excellent treatment for the female organs. Use 1 teaspoon of the leaves, roots, or both in 1 cup boiling water. Drink several cups per day. This herb may also be added to salads or soups to give nourishment.

St. John's wort is a good treatment for chronic uterus problems. Use 1 teaspoon of the powdered wort in 1 cup boiling water. Drink 3 cups per day for several weeks and then one or more cups per week to keep the female organs in tone.

Steep 1 teaspoon each of pit root and fennel seed in 1 pint boiling water for 20 minutes to make an excellent douche for inflammation of the vagina or uterus. Use only cooled mixture.

Manzanita is helpful for all female disorders. Do not use if pregnant. Use ½ teaspoon herb to 1 cup boiling water. Steep for 5 minutes and strain. Drink 1 or 2 cups per day.

Licorice is a good source of the female hormone, estrogen. This hormone helps to build the endocrine glands and is especially helpful in post hysterectomy care. Use only pure licorice made into a tea or eaten as 'candy'. Take daily.

Dong kwei is the female equivalent of ginseng (which women should not take) and it helps to stimulate the female glands and helps retard aging. Take about ½ teaspoon twice a month.

Blue flag helps stop leucorrhia which is a white, fluid vaginal discharge. Use 10-20 drops of the juice from fresh leaves to ½ cup water. Take 3 times a day. When using the powdered herb, use 1 ounce blue flag to 1 pint of water.

Oakbark tea mixed with alum helps to stop leucorrhia discharge. Use 1 teaspoon oakbark, 2 teaspoons alum and 1 cup boiling water. Sip slowly, 1-2 cups per day. Continue as needed.

The female hormone, progesterone, is contained in sarsaparilla. Progesterone helps the functioning of the ovaries and is necessary for reproduction. Use 1 teaspoon sarsaparilla to 1 cup boiling water to make a tea. Drink 1-3 cups a day as needed.

Cramps
☆Menstrual cramps have many causes, but usually indicate a lack of calcium and magnesium in the system and a negative frame of mind. Eat fresh, raw parsley or drink parsley tea. This herb helps to warm the body and supply needed vitamins and minerals.

Camomile tea is an excellent remedy for cramps as it soothes stomach tension and relaxes the nerves. Use 1 teaspoon camomile flowers to 1 cup boiling water and sip slowly as often as necessary.

Peppermint and alfalfa teas are both good to ease the discomfort of labor contractions. Use 1 teaspoon herb to 1 cup boiling water and drink as often as needed.

To Increase Menstrual Flow
Squawvine is an excellent tea which is good for the uterus and helps increase the menstrual flow. Make a strong tea from the berries and use ½ cup four times a day.

Suppressed Menstruation
Irregularity of the menstrual cycle can be caused by deficiencies of iron or calcium, excessive stress, change of climate or environment, and even your diet. A lack of B vitamins, especially B_{12} can delay menstruation. Here are some teas which assist menstruation. Women who are pregnant should avoid these herbs as they may cause miscarriages.

Pennyroyal tea helps suppressed menses. Take 1 teaspoon pennyroyal to 1 cup boiling water. Drink a cup of the warm tea every three hours.

Make a tea using ginger leaves and drink to assist menstruation. Use ¼ teaspoon ginger to 1 cup boiling water. Honey may be added if necessary. Steep 5 minutes and drink two cups per day.

☆Tansy is excellent for promoting menstrual flow. Use 1 ounce tansy to 1 pint boiling water. Steep several minutes and drink 4-5 cups per day.

Sweet basil, taken hot, is good for suppressed menses. Take 1 teaspoon herb to 1 cup boiling water. Drink 1 cup every three hours.

To assist menstruation, mix ½ ounce each of black hellborn root, mugwort, wormseed and valerian herb. Take 1 pinch of this mixture to 1 cup boiling water and steep for 5 minutes. Take ½ cup twice a day.

Cottonroot is helpful for bringing on menstruation. Use 2 ounces powdered root to 1 pint boiling water. Drink 2-3 cups per day.

Birthwort helps induce menstruation and will stimulate delivery of afterbirth. Use 1 teaspoon powdered birthwort in 1 small wineglass of white wine. Sip slowly before bedtime.

Rosemary is well known for promoting menstruation. Use 1 teaspoon herb to 1 cup boiling water and drink 1 cup warm tea every three hours.

Black cohosh, taken 5-6 grains per day, will help to stimulate menstrual flow.

Excessive Menstruation

Shepherd's purse has been known to stop bleeding within 15 minutes as it contains vitamin K. This treatment is excellent for all kinds of hemorrhages. Use 1 teaspoon herb to 1 cup boiling water and steep for several minutes. Take 1 cup as often as needed.

Rushes help to stop excessive bleeding of menstruation. Use 1 teaspoon of the root and steep 5-10 minutes in 1 cup boiling water. Drink at least 3 cups.

For prolonged menses, press the inside of the leg five inches below the knee on both legs at the same time. This will help to stop bleeding anywhere in the body within minutes. (See diagram 14).

Menopause

Hot flashes indicate that the body lacks hormones. This can be remedied by eating hormone foods daily. Cucumbers, licorice, and sarsaparilla are all high in female hormones.

Passion flower helps to soothe the body during menopause. Use 10-20 drops per day of the liquid extract from the fresh leaves or, if using powder, use 3 grains twice a day.

Miscarriages

Miscarriages are caused by a lack of amino acids in the system. Raspberry leaf tea is rich in vitamins A, B, C, G, F and minerals such as calcium, phosphorus and iron, to help prevent miscarriage. Use 1 ounce of the leaves to 1 pint of boiling water and steep for 20 minutes. Sweeten only with honey and drink 10-20 ounces per day. Raspberry leaf tea also helps one to have an easier delivery.

Infertility

Infertility occurs when the body does not have sufficient nutrients to support pregnancy. Dolomite (calcium and magnesium) helps to insure fertility in women. Eat foods which are high in calcium and magnesium or take daily supplements.

Breast Remedies
Vitamin E helps to restore sagging breasts. Daily exercise and a healthy diet are also important.

Breast cancer or cysts can be treated by using the diets recommended in the cancer section.

Running sores on the breasts indicate that the bowels are in poor condition. Place a potato poultice on the breasts and change when dry to help draw out the infection. See the digestion section for a cleansing diet to accompany this treatment.

For caked breasts, steep comfrey roots and leaves in warm water and apply in a poultice to the breasts. Drink the liquid from the steeped herbs and repeat when dry. This will help to soften caked breasts and relieve the soreness and pain.

Pregnancy and Birth
There are many good birthing books on the market and I heartily recommend home birth. Be sure you check with your naturopathic doctor before and during pregnancy.

☆ From conception to birthing, raspberry tea should be taken daily. This herb contains vitamins A, C, B, G, and E and calcium, phosphorus, iron and other nutrients which help to prevent miscarriages and ease delivery. Use 1 ounce of the leaves to 1 pint boiling water and steep for 20 minutes. Drink 10-20 ounces daily throughout pregnancy. Sip slowly.

Squawvine tea, made 1 ounce herb to 1 pint boiling water, is also helpful to the body for nutritive benefits during pregnancy. Take 2-3 glasses per day.

Pregnant women and nursing mothers should not eat the following foods as they cause gas and colic in the mother and, consequently, the baby: garlic, cauliflower, cabbage, onions, broccoli, and excess quantities of beans.

Cramps in the legs and feet during pregnancy may indicate a deficiency of vitamins B and D. These vitamins should be taken in foods and in supplement form.

During labor, have the mother suck on ice cubes or sip liquids made of peppermint, alfalfa and /or raspberry teas. These teas give liquid nourishment to the mother and help to ease tension. Liquids lost in birthing should be replaced. Drink plenty of liquids, especially if giving birth on a hot day.

Morning Sickness

Knotgrass tea helps to strengthen the womb and control nausea. Use 1 teaspoon of the herb to 1 cup boiling water. Steep 3-5 minutes and sip 1-2 cups per day.

During pregnancy, take fruit or fruit juice first in the morning to cleanse the stomach. One half hour later, eat bran, barley or other foods which are high in B-complex vitamins.

Pregnant women should make sure the bowels are clean as this will help to control nausea and protect the fetus against toxins from body wastes. See the section on digestion for more information.

Nursing

Saw palmetto promotes proper functioning of the mammary glands. Take 3-5 berries daily during the last month of pregnancy and while nursing.

Nursing mothers need extra vitamins E, B-complex and lecithin. Supplements should be taken daily.

Avocadoes supply many nutrients needed by the nursing mother. Eat an avocado daily.

☆To prepare for nursing, a mother should sip a cup of alfalfa tea daily before each feeding to insure a sufficient supply of milk. This tea also supplies many nutrients.

After a birth, the mother should drink plenty of comfrey tea, especially if stiches were made. Comfrey will help repair the episiotomy. Use 1 teaspoon comfrey root, leaves or both to 1 cup boiling water. Steep 5 minutes and take 3-5 cups per day. Use a poultice of comfrey on the incision.

To avoid tearing during birth, the opening to the vagina should be oiled with sesame seed oil daily during pregnancy to promote elasticity. Sesame oil, if rubbed over the entire body daily during pregnancy, will help prevent stretch marks and allow the skin to stretch comfortably.

After the incision has healed, the mother should drink pennyroyal tea daily to help draw the uterus and other organs back into place. Use 1 teaspoon herb to 1 cup boiling water, steep 3 minutes, strain and drink 2-3 cups per day. Continue for at least one week.

GLANDULAR SYSTEM

The glandular system maintains the tone of the body by producing many different hormones and maintaining a balance between them. The glandular system is composed of the thyroid, parathyroid, adrenal, pituitary and endocrine glands. If there is a malfunction in the glandular system, the body will feel sluggish and run down. To stimulate the system and cleanse it of impurities, massage the spots on the feet that correspond to the glands, as indicated in the foot section (diagrams 6 and 7). If these spots are tender for no external reason, it is an indication that the glands need to be stimulated.

Thyroid Gland

The following conditions may indicate that the thyroid is underfunctioning: feeling cold all the time, low energy, poor growth and, in extreme cases, an arrhythmic heartbeat.

Dulse is the best thyroid stimulant and should be taken every day to insure proper functioning of this gland. Use dulse instead of salt in soups, cereals, and whenever liquids are being cooked. One-half to one teaspoon dulse, taken daily, will sufficiently feed the thyroid and help insure vitality and normal growth.

To stimulate the thyroid, combine 2 ounces Irish moss with 2 quarts cold water and let stand overnight. In the morning bring to a boil, and simmer for 10 minutes or until the mixture is reduced to 1 quart liquid. Strain into a glass and take 1 tablespoon each morning for 3 weeks.

Pennyroyal leaves and flowers will help to restore the thyroid system. Make into a tea using 1 teaspoon leaves to 1 cup boiling water and add honey to give more nutrients. Drink 2-3 cups daily.

Ginger root stimulates the thyroid as well as the parathyroid glands and helps to produce saliva. Use ½ teaspoon freshly grated ginger root or ¼ teaspoon powder to 1 cup boiling water. Drink ½ cup twice a day.

Bugle will help to reduce enlargement of the thyroid gland. Use 1 ounce bugle to 1 pint boiling water. Drink 3 ounces 5-6 times a day. This helps to improve the appetite.

Mushrooms are helpful for all conditions of the thyroid. Eat in salads or use in cooking.

Gland Stimulants and Cleansers

To stimulate the glandular system, eat dark fruit such as grapes and blueberries and drink their juices.These juices and fruits help to build red blood cells and improve the cleansing functions of the glands.

Protein foods help to stimulate the adrenal system. Seeds, nuts, lentils and beans are good sources of protein.

Cayenne pepper, taken in small amounts of 5-7 grains, will help boost a sluggish system. The pepper may be combined with hot or cold water. Larger quantities will irritate the mucous membranes of the digestive system.

Three to five berries of saw palmetto, taken daily, will help to improve the activity of the glands.

To restore hormonal balances eliminate all white flours, sugars, and processed foods from the diet. Eat raw, fresh vegetables and plenty of fruit.

Cucumbers will stimulate hormone production. Eat daily in salads or as a snack.

Figs help to feed the hormonal system. For one day a week, eat only tree ripened figs and raw vegetable salads made with a lemon and apple juice dressing. This helps to re-establish the body rhythm and supply natural B vitamins.

Combine ½ cup sesame seeds, ¼ cup wheatgerm, and 3 tablespoons dark honey. Powder the seeds and mix the ingredients together to make small bars. Eat 2-3 small bars daily to stimulate and cleanse the glandular system.

Soy products supply the glandular system with nutrients.

To cleanse the glands, eat nothing but watermelon for 1 day. This diet is especially good during very hot weather.

Yerba mate tea, made with lemon or honey, helps to stimulate the glands and cleanse the system. Use 1 teaspoon yerba mate to 1 cup boiling water, steep 5 minutes and sip slowly.

Chickweed helps to heal the pineal and pituitary glands by supplying minerals which soothe the system. This herb helps retard aging. Eat in salads or make into a tea using 1 teaspoon chickweed to 1 cup boiling water. Drink 1-2 cups per day.

Valerian helps to eliminate poisons from the glandular system and to stimulate the glands. Use 1 teaspoon to 1 cup boiling water. Steep for 3-5 minutes and take only ½ cup per day for 1 week. Wait one month and repeat.

Combine one tablespoon flaxseed, 2 tablespoons wheat bran, 4 tablespoons rolled oats, and 1 cup vegetable broth and soak overnight. In the morning, heat the mixture and sweeten with honey. Eat slowly to help stimulate the proper functioning of the adrenal glands.

Oatstraw tea supplies minerals to the glandular system. Use 1 teaspoon oatstraw to 1 cup boiling water and steep for ½ hour. The oatstraw may be reused several times. Drink freely instead of water. This tea is especially helpful to replace mineral deficiencies created by exhaustion.

Combine equal parts carrot, celery, and radish juice with 2 tablespoons onion juice. Take 1 cup three times a day to help restore the mineral balance in the system.

Combine ½ glass fresh apple juice, ½ glass berry juice, and 4 tablespoons sesame seed oil. Drink twice a day to supply minerals and nourish the adrenal glands.

Combine 2 ounces rhubarb juice, 1 ounce beet juice and 1 ounce honey with 5 ounces water. Warm, or drink cold if the stomach is sensitive. Take daily for 1 week to restore energy.

Blend ½ cup soy milk, ½ cup lettuce juice and ½ cup celery juice together and add 2 tablespoons onion juice. Drink daily for 1 month to supply an energy booster to the body.

Mix ½ cup each soy milk and skim milk with 2 tablespoons brewer's yeast and 1 teaspoon honey. Drink daily to provide energy for the body.

HEADACHES

Headaches are caused by congestion in the system, and often it is possible to determine the location of the congestion by the characteristics of the headache. Pressure in the temples and forehead usually indicates that there is tension in the stomach, and throbbing pain often results from congestion in the liver, spleen or digestive tract. Migraine headaches are caused by excess starches and sugars in the diet. Foods that are eaten too quickly, or washed down with liquids will create gas and putrification in the stomach which can cause a headache. When an internal organ is congested, it will send signals to the brain which are interpreted as pain in the head, rather than pain from the organ. Tension is the most common cause of headaches, whether directly by affecting the brain itself, or indirectly by contributing to congestion in the system.

Aspirin is not a good remedy for headache as it cannot relieve the cause of the pain. Aspirin also deteriorates the lining of the stomach and can raise the blood pressure. The best treatment for chronic headaches is a combination of eating well, not drinking with meals, and alleviating stress. This treatment requires a little time, of course, but here are some immediate remedies for headache pain.

Headaches and Headache Pain

☆Combine ½ teaspoon fresh lemon juice and 8 ounces of water, as warm as you can drink it comfortably. Add 1 teaspoon baking soda and drink quickly while the mixture is still bubbling. In a few minutes, you will burp to expel the excess gas. Repeat every 15 minutes until the pain is gone.

For pain of headaches and to increase circulation, combine 4 parts dried rosemary, 1 part freshly ground ginger, and 2 parts honey. Make a tea using ½ cup of this mixture to 6 cups boiling water. Steep for 5 minutes, strain and drink 3 cups per day.

To help relieve headache pain, use 1 teaspoon golden seal, ¼ teaspoon dandelion root and ¼ teaspoon mandrake root in 1 pint boiling water. Steep ½ hour, strain and drink ½ cup thirty minutes before each meal.

The fresh juice of ground ivy, sniffed up the nostrils, will help releive headaches.

Basswood helps to stop headache pain. Use 1 teaspoon basswood to 1 cup boiling water and take ½ cup four times a day.

Headache Nausea

Cut 3-4 slices of fresh cucumber, place in a bowl with 1 tablespoon dried sea weed and add enough water to cover. Let the mixture stand overnight and drink the liquid first thing in the morning. This will help to remove the obstructions in the system which create nausea and headaches.

Migraine Headaches

Migraine headaches are a direct result of improper diet. Consumption of devitalized foods mades it difficult for the body to eliminate wastes efficiently. Consequently, the uneliminated wastes accumulate and block the system, making it difficult for the liver to function properly. Pancakes, waffles, pastries and other gluten foods are particularly difficult to digest. A three day cleansing fast and a subsequent diet of raw vegetables and other nutritious foods, will bring relief from migraine headaches and help to prevent their recurrance.

HEART AND CIRCULATORY SYSTEM

The heart is one of the hardest working parts of the body. Yet, as long as it functions properly, we give it little attention. Vitamins B, C, E, and dolomite help to strengthen the heart and proper exercise is vitally important. The heart functions properly if the veins and arteries of the circulatory system are kept strong and supple, and the blood is pure.

Care of the Heart

Blend the following ingredients together and drink a small 2 ounce glass 1 hour before each meal to help feed and strengthen the heart muscles and the circulatory system.

> ½ cup tomato juice
> ½ cup lemon or orange juice
> 1 tablespoon brewer's yeast
> 6 tablespoons wheat germ oil

Pour 1 quart boiling water over 1 cup fresh parsley and allow to steep for 15 minutes. Strain and refrigerate. Drink 3 cups per day as a tonic for the heart.

Angelica will relax the heart and build resistance to infections. Use ½ teaspoon angelica root powder to 1 cup boiling water. Take 2 cups daily.

Ground ivy helps to regulate the heart and cleanse the bloodstream. Take 1 teaspoon ivy in 1 cup boiling water two times per day or the equivalent amount in capsule form.

Mandrake root helps lower high blood pressure and strengthen the heart. Use ½ teaspoon root to 1 cup boiling water. Steep 3-5 minutes and drink 3 cups per day.

Oak groats are good for the heart muscles. Use in tea or grind and use in soups, stews and cooking.

Take two garlic pearlies (garlic oil in capsules) daily to help protect and strengthen the heart against circulatory diseases.

Rutin, a yellow powder made from ground buckwheat, helps to strengthen the artery walls to prevent strokes and hemorrhaging. It also makes the capillaries more supple. Take 300-500 mg daily with vitamin C.

Vitamin E helps reduce hardening of the arteries and aid healthy functioning of the circulatory system. E is found in dandelion leaves, parseley, spinach, mustard greens, turnip leaves and all green leafy vegetables. Use any of the above leaves in a blended mixture to make a good vitamin E drink.

Rosemary helps strengthen the heart. Use 1 teaspoon rosemary leaves in 1 cup boiling water, steep for 5 minutes, strain and drink three cups per day. Honey may be added if sweetening is needed.

The adrenal glands manufacture adrenalin and hormones which help tone the blood vessels and the heart. Liver, kidney, wheat germ, green leafy vegetables, soy products and yeast all stimulate the adrenal glands and the heart.

Pleurisy root is good for soothing tension in the arteries and the heart. Do not use when the skin is cold or the pulse is weak. Use 1 teaspoon pleurisy root powder in 1 cup boiling water. Take 1 cup three times a day.

Lily of the valley root is good for all heart conditions. Use the plant (not the flowers) for quieting the heart. Use ½ tablespoon herb to 1 pint boiling water. Take 1 tablespoon morning and evening. Do not exceed dosage.

☆Peppermint tea is recommended to calm the heart and relax tension around the heart. Taken daily, it is said to effectively prevent heart attacks. Use 1 teaspoon herb to 1 cup boiling water and drink freely, at least 1 cup per day.

Taking a small amount of saffron daily helps prevent artery and circulatory problems. Saffron helps rebuild tissue and prevent hardening of the arteries.

White sugar and products containing white sugar are very hard on the heart. Recent studies suggest that excessive ingestion of white sugars may cause heart problems.

Onions and garlic are good for all circulatory diseases. They reduce the possibility of heart attacks and raise the blood's capacity to prevent or dissolve clots. Use onions and garlic, boiled, fried or juiced. Eat approximately 1 clove garlic and/or ½ onion per day.

Cholesterol and the Heart

Excess cholesterol is the result of eating too many processed foods which leave gluten clogging the system. Lecithin contains phosphorus, and aids in dissolving fatty deposits in the tissues and arteries. Take at least 1 teaspoon daily or take up to 19 grains in capsule form. Some foods which are low in cholesterol are vegetable oil, fish oil, poultry without the skin, nuts, whole grain breads, gelatin, unprocessed cereals, fruits, lean meats, uncreamed cottage cheese, peanut butter, skim milk, sherbett and all vegetables.

Rapid Heart (Fibrillation)

Rapid heart may be caused by an overactive thyroid gland. This may be the result of excess toxins in the system. Make the fist into a ball with the thumb on the outside and press on the wrist of the left hand to help slow the heart and calm the tension.

The heart beat may be slowed by placing the hand over the heart and remaining quiet for several minutes. This is the natural inclination of the body after heavy exertion.

Place a compress of hot cloths on the chest to help slow the heart.

Heart Attacks

Wheat germ is very valuable for cardiac trouble, the D-alpha tocopherols it contains helps to prevent blood clots. Take 400-800 I. U. daily.

Heart attack victims should make a tight fist with the thumb on the outside. Place a hot compress on the chest to help soothe the heart and dissolve clots.

Diseases of the Heart Muscles

Place 1 pound raw unpeeled beets in an earthen jar and cover with ¼ pound pure honey and ¼ pound brown sugar. Let the mixture stand for 48 hours and take 1 tablespoon twice a day. This mixture helps to build the blood and strengthen the muscles

The following two day fast will help to relax the nervous system and restore proper functioning of the heart.

> On day one, eat nothing but one kind of fruit all day (apples, peaches, pears or berries are good). Drink at least 3 glasses of water.
> On day two, eat only brown short grain rice. Drink at least 3 glasses of water
> On day three and thereafter, eliminate all salt and sugar from the diet, continue eating normally.

Circulation

Poor circulation indicates a need for vitamins C, E, and rutin. Rutin is ground buckwheat and may be purchased at most drug counters.

To stimulate the circulation, cook the following mixture for 20 minutes or until the texture is mushy. Remove the seeds and eat 1 tablespoon each evening.

> 1 cup dates
> 1 cup figs
> ½ cup corn meal
> 3 cups water

Two or three grains of cayenne pepper, taken in a capsule or with water help the circulatory system and help prevent blood clots. Do not exceed dosage.

Bell peppers are good for the blood. Eat 1 raw bell pepper daily.

Fresh cherry juice helps to strengthen blood vessels and arteries. Drink ½ cup daily for 4 days, skip 4 days and repeat.

Queen's delight is good for cleansing and purifying the blood. Use 1/8 ounce powdered root daily in capsules or mix in fruit juice.

Spicewood bush makes a good tonic for the blood. Break up the limbs into 3" pieces and put 2-3 ounces in a double boiler. Pour 1 gallon boiling water over the herb and let the mixture steep for 1 hour. Drink 3-4 cups daily for 1 week.

To help purify the blood steep 1 tablespoon saffron flowers in 1 cup boiling water for 5 minutes, strain and place in glass or ceramic container. Take 2 tablespoons 2-3 times a day.

Sarsaparilla is a good blood purifier. Take 1 teaspoon powdered herb in 1 cup boiling water. Drink 3 cups per day.

Burdock is an excellent blood cleanser. Make a tea using 1 pint boiling water and 2 ounces burdock root. Add 3 pints cold water and boil the mixture down to 2 pints. Strain and drink 3 cups per day. Burdock may be combined with pokeroot, grapefruit, violet leaves, yellow dock, red clover, parseley or nettles.

Put the following herbs into 2 quarts cold water and boil the mixture down to 1 quart. Take 1-2 tablespoons three times a day to purify the blood.
   1 tablespoon gentian root
   1 tablespoon rhubarb
   1 tablespoon sacred bark
   1 tablespoon may apple
   1 tablespoon yellow dock
   4 tablespoons sassafras
   4 tablespoons dandelion

Sassafras is a good blood purifier. Use 1 teaspoon sassafras root or bark to 1 cup boiling water and steep for several minutes. Strain and drink 2-3 cups per day.

Dandelion root or leaves helps build up the blood and eliminate impurities. Use 1 teaspoon root or leaves to 1 cup boiling water and take 2-5 cups per day.

Peaches, eaten daily, help build up the blood and eliminate toxins in the system.

Agrimony helps to purify the blood. Take ½ teaspoon to 1 cup boiling water. Drink 3 cups per day or take the agrimony in capsules.

Blood Poisoning
Use powdered slippery elm bark and sassafras bark to treat blood poisoning. Put these herbs into a pan with as much water as will absorb and make a wet paste. Place the paste in a poultice over the affected area. This treatment is

good for poisoning from spiders, insects, snake bite, or other injuries where poison must be drawn out of the wound.

Garlic, taken raw, helps to treat blood poisoning by destroying germs in the system without harming beneficial bacteria.

Place a raw lemon over swelling caused by blood poisoning to help draw out inflammation and relieve pain. The juice of the lemon mixed with a glass of warm water and taken internally, helps to flush toxins from the system.

Varicose Veins and Arteriosclerosis
Varicose veins and arteriosclerosis result when arteries and veins lose their elasticity and become hardened. Vitamin E taken daily with two tablespoons lecithin will, over a period of two to three years, help soften veins and restore elasticity.

To strengthen capillaries and help reduce rigidity, oatstraw tea is excellent. Use 1 ounce oatstraw to 1 quart boiling water, steep for ½ hour and drink freely instead of water. Okra also contains the silicon and selenium needed to help the capillaries. Eat fresh when possible, or in soups and stews.

Arteriosclerosis responds favorably to daily supplements of garlic and vitamin E. The garlic will help restore elasticity to the hardened arteries, and the vitamin E will speed up the healing process by supplying adequate oxygen. Eat one cup of cooked garlic with fresh salads and raw vegetables. Sip plenty of water, but not within one hour of eating. Follow this diet for two consecutive days per month.

Phlebitis
Phlebitis sufferers need to drink plenty of fresh vegetable juices to help dissolve blood clots. Drinking plenty of liquids (especially water) helps to keep the system flushed out. A comfrey poultice on the outside of the affected area helps to dissolve the clot as well as comfrey tea taken internally. This diet should include only fresh juices, raw vegetables, and plenty of roughage such as greens and sprouts. Lecithin also helps to dissolve bloodclots and should be taken daily (one tablespoon). Elevate the affected area for several hours per day.

HIGH AND LOW BLOOD PRESSURE

When the circulatory system is tense, the veins and arteries constrict, creating pressure on the blood stream. Thus, tension is the cause of high blood pressure. In turn, the tension is caused by improper diet and stress. Blood pressure may be lowered by eliminating from the diet all fatty meats, spices, salt, alcohol, tobacco and white sugar. Instead, eat fresh fruits, especially fresh peaches, rolled oats, bell peppers, alfalfa, carrots, celery, parseley, bamboo shoots, zucchini squash and spinach. All of these foods help to lower blood pressure and fortify the blood.

When the blood pressure is high, the blood may break through the tiny capillaries in the nasal cavity, causing nosebleeds. This is one of the bodys' safety mechanisms to prevent internal bleeding and heart attacks. To stop a nosebleed, hold the arm on the side of the bleeding high in the air for a few moments to decrease the tension and stop the bleeding. Gently pull on the middle finger on the left or right hand until the knuckle pops. This will help to lower the blood pressure. See diagram 9.

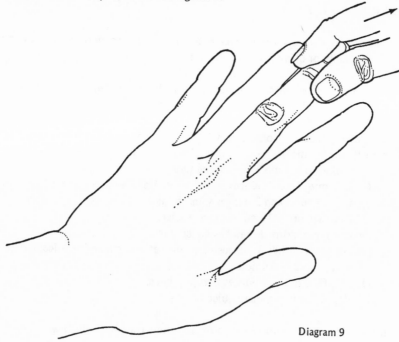

Diagram 9

High Blood Pressure

Raspberry leaf tea helps to relieve high blood pressure. Add 1 ounce of raspberry leaves to 1 pint boiling water and simmer for 20 minutes. Drink cold, 1 cup per day.

High blood pressure can be lowered by taking 1-3 garlic pearlies and vitamin E supplements daily.

Passion flowers help to control high blood pressure and to calm nervous conditions. Take three grains per day in capsule form or in tea.

☆Taking 3-4 alfalfa tablets per day will control both high and low blood pressure and build up the resistance to disease. Alfalfa will also help to strengthen the blood cells and arteries.

Asafetida will help to reduce high blood pressure. Use 1 ounce asafetida powder mixed with 1 pint boiling water. Take 1 tablespoon cooled liquid per day for adults and smaller amounts for children. Never take more than 1 tablespoon per day. Three grains of the asafetida in capsule form may be substituded for the tea.

Cucumber juice or raw, fresh, cucumbers help to lower blood pressure. Eat 1 cucumber daily or drink ½ cup of the juice.

Stinging nettles are a good treatment for high blood pressure. Use 1 teaspoon nettles to 1 cup boiling water. Take 4-5 cups per day.

The following diet is recommended for high blood pressure patients. In addition to the juices drink three 8-ounce glasses of water per day. Eat no other foods or liquids during the length of the diet

On day one, take 7 ounces carrot juice, 4 ounces celery juice, 2 ounces parseley juice and 3 ounces spinach juice.

On day two, drink 12 ounces carrot juice.

On day three, drink 9 ounces spinach juice.

On day four, drink 3 ounces each of beet and cucumber juice and 10 ounces of carrot juice.

On day five, drink 3 ounces parseley juice.

On day six, drink spinach juice all day.

Boil unpeeled potatoes for 15 minutes to produce a liquid which will help to lower blood pressure. Drink 2 cups potato water per day.

Sassafras and prickly ash will make a tea which helps to purify the blood and lower blood pressure. Use ½ teaspoon of each to 1 cup boiling water and take 2 cups per day.

Nose Bleeds

Adder's tongue is good for nosebleeds. Make a tea using 1 teaspoon adder's tongue herb to 1 cup boiling water and drink 2 cups per day.

Cayenne pepper, taken in tea, helps to improve circulation and reduce blood pressure. Use 1/12 of 1 grain in 1 cup boiling water and drink 1 cup per day. The cayenne may also be taken in capsule form. Do not exceed dosage.

Low Blood Pressure

Excess toxins in the blood are a result of nutritional deficiencies and are the primary cause of low blood pressure. Anaemia is caused by poor digestion, iron deficiency and consumption of devitalized foods. Anaemia indicates that the system is not producing enough red corpuscles. Prolonged anaemia will rob the bone marrow of corpuscles and will thereby weaken the bone. Low blood pressure (hypoglycemia) and anaemia are not the same, but they are related, and the treatments are similar. The symptoms of anaemia are: unnatural pallor, loss of strength, shortness of breath, headaches, nervousness, cold hands and feet, heart palpitations, and lack of energy. Many of these symptoms are concurrent with those of low blood pressure (hypoglycemia).

Of course the diet is very important with either condition. Foods which must be eliminated from the diet are: white sugar, flours of wheat, oats, rye and barley, and all starchy foods. Avoid all canned fruits and vegetables, coffee and non-herbal teas. In addition, eat no animal fats, butter, cream cheese, bacon, pork, duck or goose, and take only small amounts of honey. Some valuable foods are skim milk, organ meat, muscle meat, tongue, poultry, eggs and sunflower oil. Eat plenty of brown rice, corn, millet products, rice flour, corn flour and corn meal, fresh vegetables, and fresh and dried fruits. Fresh juices such as apple, grape, carrot and beet juices are particularly good. Be sure to include in your diet plenty of B and E vitamin foods as well as those high in calcium, magnesium and pantothenic acid.

To help raise blood pressure mix ½ cup soy bean powder and 1½ cups water in a blender at high speed for 3-4 minutes. Strain and drink ½ cup three times a day.

Chives will help to control low blood pressure. Eat at least ½ bunch per day.

Alfalfa is a good treatment for both high and low blood pressure as it helps fortify the blood and build up resistance to disease. Take 3-4 tablets daily.

Vitamin C will help to control the level of blood sugar. Vitamin C also provides long lasting energy. Take daily in fresh fruits and in supplemental form.

Peas are an especially good treatment for hypoglycemia as they contain vitamins A, B_1, B_6 and nicotinic acid.

☆To build red blood cells, cover 1 pound unpeeled, raw beets with ¼ pound each raw honey and brown sugar. Let stand for 48 hours and take 1 tablespoon of the mixture twice a day.

Dandelions contain natural salts which help to purify the blood by destroying acid. Dandelion is an excellent treatment for anaemia Use 1 teaspoon dandelion root or leaves to 1 cup boiling water. Steep for 30 minutes and drink 3 cups per day.

Anaemia should be treated with lots of fresh air, good nourishing foods rich in iron and minerals, and by keeping the bowels open. Prunes are an excellent source of energy, contain vitamins A, B_1, B_{12}, and C, and will promote proper functioning of the bowels.

Treat anaemia with tea made from any of these herbs: rosemary, fennel, sage, red poppy and caraway. Use 1 teaspoon herb to 1 cup boiling water. Steep 5 minutes and drink two cups per day.

INSECT BITES AND STINGS

Ants
Ants cannot and will not cross a place where garlic has been rubbed. Take a fresh raw bulb of garlic and rub onto area where ants enter. Repeat when needed.

Bee and Wasp Stings
Place wet mud on the sting, allow mud to dry and peel off. The mud draws out the stinger as it dries and helps control swelling.

Honeysuckle juice helps relieve bee stings. Repeat if necessary.

A slice of peeled raw onion placed on the sting will draw out the swelling and lessen the pain.

Wheat germ oil, applied to stings will help reduce swelling and relieve pain. Apply to sting, repeating as often as necessary.

Moisten one-third teaspoon of unseasoned meat tenderizer with 1 teaspoon water and apply to insect stings. This helps to relieve the pain and minimize allergic reactions.

Vitamins B and C, taken internally, help the body adjust to stings and bites.

Bicarbonate of soda mixed with water soothes bee stings and reduces swelling.

Basil leaves mixed with water and applied to bee or wasp stings will help to draw out the poison.

Vinegar, dabbed onto insect bites, helps to reduce pain.

Fleas and Flies
Rue helps repel flies. Make into a strong tea using 1 teaspoon rue to 1 cup boiling water, steep for 10-15 minutes and spray in the room or onto plants.

Put bay leaves in containers of grains and flours to keep out insects.

Place orange peels and cloves in a ventilated closet bag to repel moths.

Make a tea, using 1 teaspoon thyme to 1 cup boiling water and spray around windows to repel flies.

Winter savory stuffed into a pillow and placed in the sleeping quarters or into the bed will drive away fleas. Camomile flowers may be added for a more pleasing scent.

Pennyroyal, eucalyptus, rosemary and mint all help to disperse fleas and flies. They may be used separately or together by hanging the herbs in the room or by putting in pillows.

Hips of sassafras placed in a bowl of fresh fruit will eliminate fruit flies or gnats. A strong tea of sassafras sprinkled around the house will keep flies away.

Mosquitoes
Rub manzanita leaves or tea onto the body to repel mosquitoes.

Rub eucalyptus oil onto the body or add a small amount to the bath to keep mosquitoes from biting.

Citronella repels mosquitoes. Rub sparingly onto the body. Citronella has a strong scent and may cause allergic reactions.

☆ Rub powdered sandalwood onto mosquito bites to stop the itching.

Pure, fresh lemon juice relieves itching from bug bites of all kinds. Rub onto bites. Reapply when needed.

A piece of flannel dipped in spirits of camphor and hung in a room will help rid the area of mosquitoes.

Ear Mites
For mites in the ears use one drop of camphor-phenique in each ear. Wait one week and put 3-4 drops hydrogen peroxide in each ear. Mites will be washed out.

Lice
Cleanse hair with water and green soap and cut off as much of the "lice hair" as possible. Make an ointment by blending the fruit and leaves of wormwood and lanolin in a blender. Rub ointment onto affected areas to destroy lice.

Larkspur helps destroy parasitic insects. Make a tea of 1 ounce larkspur powder or leaves to 1 pint boiling water. Take 10 drops twice a day internally. Use the liquid externally on the hair and repeat 2-3 times daily until condition is cleared.

For lice, make a mixture of 2 tablespoons rue oil, 8 ounces light beer, and 1 quart tobacco water. Apply mixture to affected areas nightly for 5 nights.

Mix 1 quart tobacco water and apply to affected areas daily for 1 week to kill lice.

Scabies

Make a solution of 2 teaspoons juniper berries to 1 pint boiling water. Steep for one-half hour. After cooling, divide into four parts. Drink one part four times a day. Repeat recipe and bathe in the solution. This treatment will help relieve the itch and drive out the parasites.

Take a bath washing affected parts with green soap to open the burrows of the scabies Then make an ointment from the ingredients listed below and rub into affected areas thoroughly. Do not change underwear or bathe for three or four days. Then boil all clothes and bedclothes which have come in contact with the skin.

¼ teaspoon zinc sulfate
¼ teaspoon sulfur flowers
¼ teaspoon basillion
¼ teaspoon castor oil
¼ teaspoon gum styrax

Snakebite

For snakebite, mix tobacco with saliva or water to form a paste. Apply paste to bite and change when dry. This poultice helps draw poisons from the system.

Avens herb, when worn on the person, helps to ward off snakes.

To keep snakes away from your house, plant onions or members of the onion family nearby.

KIDNEY AND BLADDER

The kidneys and bladder are responsible for cleansing wastes from the blood and eliminating them in the form of urine. Without sufficient water, the kidneys become clogged because they cannot excrete these toxins. The residue retained in the body can cause lower back pain and inflammation of the kidneys. Foods containing vitamins A,B_2,B_6,C, E, and K will help prevent and fight diseases of the kidneys and bladder. Spinach, mangoes, nutmeg, pumpkin seeds, cucumber juice, asparagus, dandelion, grape juice, beets, carrot juice, radishes and soy lecithin are good sources of these essential vitamins. These same foods will feed the bladder and help to prevent formation of bladder and kidney stones.

☆ Kidney and Bladder Infections

Use dry curd cottage cheese in a poultice over the crotch area to help stop stinging and burning of kidney infections and draw out the inflammation. Use about 1 teaspoon cottage cheese and change the poultice 3-4 times per day. Wear day and night for two weeks or as long as needed. Throughout this treatment, drink five or more cups of comfrey or oatstraw tea per day.

Flaxseed helps to fight kidney and bladder infections. Use 3 teaspoons flaxseeds in 2 cups boiling water, steep 5 minutes and drink 2 cups every day for at least one week. If you wish to gain weight, eat the flaxseeds. If not, strain before drinking. A comfrey poultice, placed over the kidney or bladder area, will help promote recovery.

All kidney and bladder infections should be treated by massaging between the 3rd and 4th toes. This stimulates the flow of fresh blood to the organs and promotes cleansing. See diagram 6.

Juniper berries are an excellent treatment for all kidney conditions. Use several berries in 1 cup boiling water and drink 3-4 cups per day.

Buchue leaves help clear kidneys and bladder infections. Steep 1 teaspoon of the leaves in 1 cup boiling water for ½ hour. Use 1-2 cups cooled tea per day. Chewing the leaves and blossoms also will help fight infections.

Vitamins C and E are necessary for proper functioning of the kidney and bladder. A lack of these vitamins will lower natural resistance.

To Stimulate Urination

Dandelion, used in equal parts with butcher's broom herb helps to increase urination. Use ½ teaspoon each to 1 cup boiling water. Steep for 5 minutes and drink 1-2 cups per day.

Cleaver's herb helps to break up the solids in the urine and increase elimination. This herb can also help soothe irritations of the urinary tract. Make into a tea using 1 teaspoon leaves to 1 cup boiling water. Steep for 5 minutes and drink 1-2 cups per day or more as needed.

Make a tea using 1 teaspoon fresh corn silk to 1 cup boiling water, steep 3-5 minutes and drink three cups per day. This herb helps to increase the flow of urine and soothe urinary tract pain.

Boil together equal parts of horseradish and beer. Give 1 cup three times a day to stimulate urination.

Anise, caraway and sweet fennel all help to increase elimination. Use in tea or add to breads, soups, etc.

Make a strong tea using 1 heaping teaspoon squawvine to 1 cup boiling water. Steep for 20 minutes, strain and take ½ cup four times a day for urinary problems.

Manzanita, taken in a tea, is helpful for all kidney ailments. Use ½ teaspoon herb to 1 cup boiling water and steep for 10 minutes. Strain and drink 2 cups per day.

For bladder or kidney obstructions and vertigo, make a tea using ½ teaspoon each of vervain and dandelion to 1 cup boiling water. Steep for 10 minutes and drink 1-2 cups per day.

Birch bark and leaves help increase the flow of urine. Make a tea using 1 teaspoon leaves or bark to 1 cup boiling water. Steep for 10 minutes and drink 1-2 cups per day.

Juniper berries help soothe irritation of the urinary tract and increase the flow of urine. Use 1 teaspoon of the berries to 1 cup boiling water. Steep until cool, strain and drink slowly. Juniper berries give the urine a violet-like smell.

Bedwetting
One teaspoon of pure unfiltered honey at bedtime helps the body to retain water and promotes sound sleep.

Plaintain, St. John's wort, corn silk, fennel seeds, buchue and milkweed are all herbs which help prevent bedwetting. Use any one of these herbs to make a tea using 1 teaspoon herb to 1 cup boiling water. Steep 5 minutes, strain and sip slowly just before bedtime.

Too Frequent Urination
When too frequent urination is a problem, use mouse ear leaves. This herb helps soothe the irritation and cleanse the kidneys and bladder. Use 1 handful mouse ear leaves to 1 pint boiling water, steep 5 minutes, strain and take ½

cup four times a day. Treatment should continue for 1 month to prevent recurrence. The following herbs may be substituted for the mouse ear: marshmallow root, or rocky mountain grape root.

Kidney and Gall Stones and Gravels

Kidney and gall stones are small "balls" formed by excess cholesterol which the body was unable to eliminate. Care should be taken to reduce cholesterol foods from the diet. Eat plenty of raw, fresh vegetables and vegetables juices. Cleaver's herb helps to break up the cholesterol deposits and should be taken daily. Use 1 teaspoon cleaver's herb to 1 cup boiling water. Steep 10 minutes and drink cooled tea.

Vitamin C, taken daily, will help to break up the cholesterol and dissolve the stones.

Lecithin helps to dissolve cholesterol deposits in the body. Take 1 teaspoon daily in capsule, crystal or liquid form.

☆Take camomile tea daily for 2 weeks to help break up stones and pass them through the urinary tract and out of the body. Make a tea using 1 teaspoon camomile to 1 cup boiling water. Drink 5-7 cups per day. I have seen kidney and gall stones dissolve completely in one week with this treatment. One particular patient had been scheduled for surgery, but by the end of the week, surgery was unnecessary.

If kidney or gall stones are of long standing and are painful, lie down on the floor and slowly sip ½ cup warm olive oil. The stones will pass through the body quickly. The warm oil helps to open the ducts and allow the passage of the stones or gravels. Repeat up to three times, if necessary.

Dandelion helps to cleanse the gall bladder and dissolve stones. Use 1 teaspoon dandelion leaves or root to 1 cup boiling water or eat raw dandelion in salads.

Pear juice helps cleanse the gall bladder and restore proper functioning. Drink slowly, several cups per day.

Trailing arbutis is a good treatment for gravels and all diseases of the urinary tract. Use 1 teaspoon to 1 cup boiling water and steep for 3-5 minutes. Sip slowly, 2-3 cups per day.

LIVER AND SPLEEN

A healthy, well functioning liver is necessary to the well being of every part of the body. The liver inspects, and when necessary processes assimilated foods and distributes them throughout the body. The liver regulates the balance of water and salt in the system, and extracts and stores sugars, fats, and some vitamins. The bile which is produced by the liver is necessary for healthy formation and maintainance of the bones. The liver also helps to control bleeding and is involved in the production of sex hormones. Obviously, an unhealthy liver will have a detrimental effect on every part of the body, but a proper diet will keep this important organ functioning properly. The spleen works with the liver to distribute blood throughout the body. The spleen also forms and stores blood cells and destroys and eliminates unnecessary blood cells through the liver.

A sallow complexion indicates that there is congestion in the liver. Loss of appetite, chronic bowel problems, and spots on the hands, arms and face are other indications that the liver is not functioning properly.

Vitamins B and C are particularly valuable for treating liver malfunctions. Raw carrots, carrot juice, grapes, parseley, limes, wild yams, bell peppers, nuts, parsnips, spinach and beets are all high in these vitamins and help to cleanse the liver and spleen.

Liver Cleansers

Drink one 3 ounce glass of black cherry juice every third morning for one month. Sip the juice at least ½ hour before eating or drinking anything else.

☆Parseley, boiled in water, helps clear liver obstructions. Make a tea using 1 teaspoon parseley to 1 cup boiling water. Make 4 cups per day to help dissolve obstructions of the liver.

Carrot juice is an excellent liver cleanser as it stimulates the system to eliminate wastes. If the skin begins to turn yellow while carrot juice is being taken, it indicates that the liver is congested Continue drinking the carrot juice. In 1-2 days the skin should regain a normal appearance as the liver is cleansed.

Raspberry leaves help clear liver congestion. Use 1 ounce of the leaves in ½ pint boiling water. Simmer for 20 minutes and drink cold. Take 2-3 cups throughout the day. Continue treatment for 3-5 days.

Steep the leaves and stems of the strawberry plant in boiling water for 5-10 minutes. Use 1 ounce of the leaves to 1 pint boiling water and drink 2-3 glasses per day.

Drink one cup raw beet juice first thing in the morning to stimulate and help cleanse the liver. Sip slowly and do not repeat for several days.

Pure apple juice helps to cleanse the liver and is beneficial in all liver conditions. Drink freely.

Dandelion root will help to stimulate and cleanse the liver and reduce swelling of the pancreas and spleen. Toast dandelion root in the oven and grind. Use 1 teaspoon to 1 cup boiling water. Brew like coffee, and sweeten with honey.

Make a tea using 10-20 drops of blue flag juice in ½ cup boiling water or use 1 ounce powdered herb to 1 pint boiling water. This tea will help to cleanse the liver and restore proper functioning. Drink three cups per day.

Use the following diet for five days to treat all liver conditions. Do not take any other foods or liquids, except for water.

> On day one, drink 10 ounces carrot juice, 3 ounces beet juice and 3 ounces cucumber juice.
>
> On day two, drink 10 ounces of carrot juice and 10 ounces of spinach juice.
>
> On day three, drink 16 ounces carrot juice.
>
> On day four, drink 2 ounces coconut juice, 3 ounces beet juice and 11 ounces carrot juice.
>
> On day five, drink 2 ounces celery juice, 2 ounces parseley juice, and 9 ounces carrot juice.

To help rejuvenate the liver, make a tea using 1 teaspoon each of dandelion root, angelica, wormwood and gentian. Simmer the herbs together with 2 cups boiling water and steep for 10 minutes. Add 2 quarts apple juice and 4 ounces freshly squeezed lemon juice. Drink in small portions, about 4 ounces at a time, for 2-3 days. During these days, eat only stewed apples or drink pure apple juice. Repeat once a month.

Combine 4 ounces hawthorne, 2 ounces each of balm leaves and red sage, and 1 ounce each of cardamon, cinnamon, and saffron. Steep these herbs in 2 quarts cold water for 24 hours. Add 4 ounces of honey, strain and drink 2-3 cups per day. This will help to reduce swelling of the spleen and stimulate production of blood cells.

Itching from Bile Retention

When cleansing the liver the body may itch. This is a reaction from the elimination of excess bile. To help alleviate this condition, drink a glass of water with the juice of ½ lemon in it. Drink this liquid as warm as possible, first thing in the morning.

Jaundice (Hepatitis)

Jaundice, commonly called hepatitis, develops when the liver is producing too much bile. This excess bile causes the skin to turn yellow. Infectious hepatitis is contagious, but as a rule a healthy liver will not contract the disease. Hepatitis (jaundice) can also be caused by severe inflammation of the liver due to an imbalance within the organ. This is a very serious condition which must be treated immediately. If ignored, the liver can be permanently damaged. Cleansing the liver regularly will prevent this type of inflammation. If you should contract jaundice, the following treatments are beneficial.

☆To treat jaundice (hepatitis) when the patient is exhibiting the symptoms or turning "yellow". Combine ½ cup each of tomato juice and sauerkraut juice. Drink 8 ounces of the combined juices three times a day and do not eat. Drink plenty of water. Continue daily until all symptoms are gone and the normal pigmentation is restored.

Mix ½ cup tomato juice and ½ cup citrus juice with 6 tablespoons wheat germ oil in a blender and drink 1 glass three times per day. Sip the mixture slowly and take 1 hour after each meal. If jaundice (hepatitis) is severe, eliminate foods or eat only fresh, raw salads with lemon juice and olive oil dressing.

Agrimony is helpful for liver ailments including jaundice. Use 1 ounce herb to 1 pint boiling water. Steep 5 minutes, strain and drink ½ cup twice a day.

When nausea accompanies jaundice, mix small amounts of powdered golden seal root with water. Taking this mixture helps to supply nourishment and to control the nausea.

When jaundice is contracted in conjunction with another disease, such as gonorrhea, drink only hot water for the first three days. Thereafter, drink boxleaf tea made from boxleaf hedge using 1 ounce leaves to 1 pint water.

Take as warm as possible. Slowly sip throughout the day. Continue until condition improves and energy is restored.

Wall flowers help to control jaundice. Make into a tea using 1 teaspoon to 1 cup boiling water. Steep for 3-5 minutes and strain. Drink 4 cups per day.

Dodder is an effective treatment for diseases of the spleen. Use in a tea made with 1 teaspoon dodder to 1 cup boiling water. Steep 3-5 minutes and strain. Drink 3 cups per day.

Ground ivy helps the spleen to function properly. Make a tea using 1 teaspoon ivy to 1 cup boiling water and drink 2 cups per day.

May apple helps to stimulate the discharge of bile Use 1 teaspoon herb to 1 pint boiling water. Steep several minutes, strain, and take 1 teaspoon twice a day.

Diabetes

Diabetes is a serious condition caused by the failure of the pancreas to produce sufficient quantities of insulin. This lack on insulin throws the body into shock. It is very dangerous and, if not treated immediately, can be fatal. The diabetic must replenish the system with the necessary nutrients and avoid starches and sugars until the pancreas and spleen can handle their metabolism. Jerusalem artichokes, string beans, almonds, wild yams, and dandelion will help stimulate the production of insulin. These herbs and vegetables contain high concentrations of vitamins B and C. Vitamin C helps to reduce the need for insulin and should be taken in large doses by the diabetic. All soy products will help to restore proper functioning of the pancreas. Diabetes is not an "incurable" disease, and with proper diet and nutrition, it can be brought under control. The following diet, followed closely for 5-6 months or longer, will help restore the natural functioning processes of the pancreas and spleen.

On the first day, drink 7 ounces carrot juice, 4 ounces celery juice, 2 ounces parsley juice and 3 ounces spinach juice.

On the second day, drink 10 ounces carrot juice and 8 ounces spinach juice.

On the third day, drink 7 ounces carrot juice, 5 ounces lettuce juice, and 4 ounces cucumber juice.

On the fourth day, drink 7 ounces carrot juice, 5 ounces celery juice, 2 ounces endive juice, and 3 ounces parsley juice.

On the fifth day, drink 9 ounces carrot juice, 5 ounces celery juice, and 2 ounces parsley juice.

On the sixth day, drink 6 ounces carrot juice, 5 ounces brussel sprout juice, and 5 ounces string bean juice.

On the seventh day, begin again with day one and continue the order.

Other than the juices, eat only raw salads with lemon juice and olive oil dressing and 2 or more glasses of water daily. This diet provides all the necessary nutrients.

Bitter root is good for diabetes because it helps to stimulate the pancreas. Use 1 teaspoon root to 1 cup boiling water. Drink 3 cups per day.

Yarrow contains some of the same active ingredients as insulin and, as such, is very beneficial for diabetics. Make a tea using 1 teaspoon of the flowers to 1 cup boiling water. Drink 4 cups per day for six months. Eat three Jerusalem artichokes per day in conjunction with the yarrow tea.

Huckleberry leaves are a good treatment for diabetes. Steep 1 ounce leaves in 1 quart boiling water for 4 hours. Drink three glasses per day.

Dandelion contains many vitamins and minerals, and is perhaps the best overall herb for diabetics. Diabetics should eat the fresh greens in salads and drink 3-4 cups of the tea daily. Make the tea using 1 teaspoon dandelion leaves or root to 1 cup boiling water and steep for 5 minutes. Strain and sip slowly.

Balm helps to stimulate the liver, kidneys and spleen and is a good treatment for diabetes. Make a tea using 1 teaspoon balm leaves to 1 cup boiling water. Drink 2-3 cups per day.

Bananas are particularly good for diabetics because they are easily metabolized and have high nutritional value.

Cirrhosis of the Liver

Cirrhosis is caused by a build up of toxins in the body which break down the filtering system of the liver and impede the production of red blood cells. Alcohol, tobacco and chemicals, including pollutants from the air, pass through the liver and tax its cleansing mechanisms. The best treatment for this condition is a strict diet designed to give the liver nutrition which is easily assimilated and to help stop the deterioration. Parsnips and all the foods previously mentioned for the liver are helpful.

This diet, taken in order and repeated until the condition clears, will help to restore the natural rhythm to the liver. The causes of the condition: alcohol, tobacco, chemicals, etc. must be eliminated in order to complete the recovery of the organ. In addition to the juices listed below, raw salads may be eaten using lemon juice and olive oil as dressing. Other foods should be avoided but liquids such as comfrey tea, alfalfa tea or teas recommended in the liver section may be used.

On day one, drink 7 ounces carrot juice, 4 ounces celery juice, 2 ounces parseley juice and 3 ounces spinach juice.

On day two, drink 10 ounces carrot juice and 6 ounces spinach juice.

On day three, drink 10 ounces carrot juice, 3 ounces beet juice and 3 ounces cucumber juice.

On day four, drink 8 ounces carrot juice, 5 ounces lettuce juice and 3 ounces spinach juice.

On day five, drink 1 pint grapefruit juice.

MALE PROBLEMS

Males need iron, dolomite and magnesium in large quantities. The predominance of all disorders related to the male organs can be helped by these minerals plus vitamin E. Pumpkin seeds and cucumbers are high sources of both vitamins, minerals and male hormones. Men should eat up to one pound of pumpkin seeds per day or 1-2 cucumbers.

For all Male Problems
Massage the back of the leg behind the ankle to treat all infections or other male problems. Massaging this part of the leg will help to soothe the organs, relax tension, and stimulate proper circulation to the male organs. See diagram 10.

Prostate Gland Disorders
Enlarged prostate has been successfully treated with magnesium Take dolomite and vitamin D. Three 200mg tablets per day.

Urinary disorders of the prostate gland may be treated by soaking 2 tablespoons juniper berries overnight in 1 ounce water. In the morning, add 1 pint boiling water and steep for ½ hour. Drink one cup morning and evening for two days.

☆Pumpkin seeds are an effective treatment for disorders of the prostate caused by a lack of male hormones. They are high in phosphorus, iron, vitamins A, B, and calcium and are high in protein and unsaturated fat.

Prostate trouble indicates a lack of male hormones. One or two cucumbers eaten daily will help to feed the glands.

Bruised melliot leaves, made into a poultice with camomile will help to reduce inflammation of the prostate gland.

Watercress makes an excellent poultice for the prostate. Use to decrease inflammation of the gland.

Vitamin E is a hormone which energizes and lubricates the male sex glands. Vitamin E is found in wheat germ, unhulled breads, green leafy vegetables, cucumbers, pumpkin seeds, peas, beets, nuts, and egg yolks.

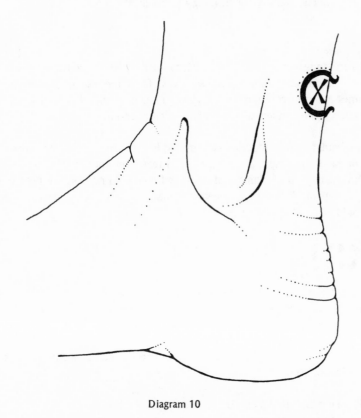

Diagram 10

Bruised or Swollen Scrotum
Bruised scrotum can be relieved by using a comfrey poultice on the scrotum to draw out the inflammation and reduce swelling and soreness. Comfrey tea should be drunk freely. Use 1 teaspoon leaves or root to 1 cup boiling water.

Impotency
Oatstraw tea supplies silicon and selenium to the system to help restore potency. Use 2 teaspoons herb to 1 cup boiling water and drink freely. Oatstraw may be re-used several times and will remain strong.

Calcium and magnesium deficiencies can decrease potency. Supplemental vitamins can help restore potency. The diet must be balanced, as any deficiency will impede healthy functioning of the glands.

Sterility
Hare lettuce and sowthistle will help restore fertility. Steep 1½ heads hare lettuce in ½ gallon pure alcohol for two days. Take 1 ounce of the mixture three times a day in conjunction with a high hormone diet. Eat plenty of cucumbers and green peppers which contain calcium and magnesium.

Ginseng stimulates the endocrine system and is a source of male hormones. It should be taken sparingly, approximately ¼ teaspoon once or twice a month. Men who eat beef, pork, lamb and other red meats do not usually need this further stimulant. Vegetarians, however, may use ginseng effectively. This herb should not be taken by women.

SKIN

Skin eruptions usually indicate that one of the elimination processes is not functioning properly. This malfunction could be located in the intestinal tract, the kidney and bladder system, or in the glandular system. Skin eruptions can also be caused by external irritations from poison oak, ivy, nettles and parasites. Some naturopathic solutions to specific skin problems are given on the following pages.

Acne, Blackheads, Pimples and Blemishes
Yarrow root tea is an excellent face wash to help control acne. Use 1 teaspoon yarrow root in 1 cup boiling water. Steep 5 minutes, strain and use cooled mixture several times a day.

For blackheads and oily skin, mix ½ cup non-alkaline soap with ¼ cup each of cornmeal and almond meal. Keep the mixture in a closed container, and use once or twice a day when washing the face. Dip a wet sponge or cloth into the mixture and rub the face. Allow the mixture to dry on the skin before rinsing the face with warm water, then with cool water. Blot the skin dry. This mixture helps to dislodge oil and dust embedded in the skin.

☆ One green pepper, one carrot and one stalk of celery eaten daily for lunch will help to clear up acne and clean the digestive tract.

Apricots, eaten daily, will help to control acne and pimples.

To help clear up acne, take vitamins A, E and brewer's yeast daily and apply peppermint oil to the affected area. Repeat daily for one month using only organic products.

Comfrey contains allentoin which helps to clear many skin conditions. Make a tea using 1 teaspoon comfrey leaves or root and 1 cup boiling water, steep for 5 minutes, strain and drink 3-4 cups per day.

Blackheads and open sores indicate that the bowels are in bad condition. Treat the bowel functions and rub lemon juice on the face each night. Wait until morning to wash the lemon juice from the face.

For all skin disorders, combine 2 ounces red clover, 1 ounce of burdock,1 ounce of blue flag and ½ ounce sassafras with 1 pint cold water. Allow the mixture to stand overnight. In the morning, bring the mixture to a boil and simmer slowly for 15-20 minutes. When cool, strain and drink 1½ ounces three times a day until the condition improves.

Brown rice contains many amino acids and, consequently, is good for all skin conditions.

Violet leaf tea is good for all skin diseases. Use 1 teaspoon leaves to 1 cup boiling water. Drink three cups per day.

To help control all skin diseases, drink one quart of fresh juice per day.

Pimples and other spots on the face will respond well to a treatment of watercress leaves. Watercress helps prevent vitamin deficiencies which affect the skin. Use the fresh leaves in salads for sources of vitamins A, B_1, B_2, C, iron, magnesium, copper and a lot of calcium.

For pimples and boils, use the birch tree bark. Make a tea using 1 cup of bark in 1 quart of boiling water. Boil mixture together for a few minutes, cool, and strain. Drink the mixture throughout the day instead of water. Continue until the condition improves.

Cucumber juice, applied externally, will help to heal skin eruptions. Drinking the juice helps to treat the internal causes of skin diseases.

The roots and leaves of avens herb, make into a tea or poultice, will help to clear the skin of freckles and eruptions.

Soapwort herb aids the healing of skin diseases. The powdered herb mixed with water can be applied externally. Repeat daily as needed.

To help clear acne conditions, make a tea using equal parts of queen's delight and bittersweet herb. One teaspoon of the combined herbs to 1 cup boiling water. Drink freely during the day.

All skin conditions can be improved by fasting and then eating properly after the body has been cleansed.

Bloodblisters indicate that the blood vessels are weak. Take oatstraw and dandelion tea daily to help strengthen the blood vessels and supply oxygen. Use ½ teaspoon each to 1 cup boiling water and drink three or more cups per day. Eat fresh okra and plenty of fruits.

Athlete's Foot and Fungus

For athlete's foot, dab vinegar onto affected areas in the morning and evening and soak the socks in vinegar and let dry before using. Wipe the shoes with vinegar to help kill the fungus.

To help clear athlete's feet and fungus, boil 1 cup clover blossoms with water until mixture thickens. When the pulp has cooled, dab onto the affected part of the dry feet. Repeat nightly until condition improves.

Campho-phenique powder rubbed into the affected area, will help to kill fungus infections.

Make a tea using crushed green walnut hulls. Drink freely to help kill fungus anywhere in the body.

Combine equal parts of blackberry leaves, marigold flowers, raw currant juice and elder blossoms to make a paste mixture. Rub this mixture into the skin, let dry, and rub the skin with a closely woven cloth bag filled with oatmeal. This helps to scrub off any loose flakes of skin.

For any foot infection, wash the socks every day with green soap and rinse with vinegar to help kill the bacteria.

For athlete's foot and fungus, crush together 2 teaspoons riboflavin, 3 teaspoons niacin, 2 teaspoons pantothenic acid and 2 teaspoons brewer's yeast powder and mix with 2 teaspoons sesame seed oil. Apply mixture once a day to the affected area, particularly between the toes and on the nails. Put on a pair of clean socks to keep the mixture on the feet. Scrub the feet once a day to remove skin flakes and reapply mixture after drying the feet throughly. Store remainder of the mixture in the refrigerator and add more sesame oil if the mixture is too thick to apply.

Bed Sores and Old Sores
Combine catnip, brewer's yeast, and whole wheat bread with 1 tablespoon milk and boil the mixture to a mush. When cooled, bind the mixture onto the skin with a clean cloth. Change when dry, replacing the cloth each time with a clean one.

Boils
☆To help draw a boil to a head, apply a poultice of chopped garlic. Repeat until the swelling has been drawn out. Do not lace the boil as this may help spread the infection.

Bruises and Wounds
Bruising easily indicates that the body may have a need for silicon, vitamin C or rutin. Oatstraw tea helps to supply silicon and fresh fruits and fruit juices to supply vitamin C. Rutin is found in ground buckwheat and may be purchased at most drug counters.

Mix equal quantities of lard and salt together and apply externally to bruised areas to stimulate circulation and replace damaged cells.

Witch hazel bark and leaves, in poultice form, helps to heal bruises. Change the poultice several times a day.

For proud flesh, or skin that peels off repeatedly, combine ½ ounce each of poppy seeds and camomile into a bottle with 1 pint boiling water. Apply externally, one teaspoon at a time, several times a day.

Make a paste of equal parts charcoal and wholewheat flour mixed with water or spittle. Use the paste in a poultice on proud flesh. Change the poultice when dry and continue until condition improves.

Burns, Sunburn
The toxic effects of sunburn may be reduced by taking vitamin D. This vitamin is also helpful for sunstroke.

For sunburn pain, make an ointment of plantain leaves and lanolin. This mixture also helps to keep the skin youthful.

☆The juice of the aloe vera plant will help relieve the pain from burns of all kinds. Apply as often as necessary. This juice also helps stop scarring.

For burns, use a comfrey poultice made with comfrey leaves and vaseline or oil rubbed into the surface of the cloth to keep the poultice from sticking.

Skin Cancer
Castor oil or comfrey, applied in an external poultice, will help to draw out cancerous tissue. Change the poultice when dry. As part of the same treatment, drink 5-6 cups comfrey tea per day. See the cancer section for additional information.

Golden seal root, made into a tea and used as a wash is helpful for all diseases of the skin.

To remove skin growths, use the herb cancerillo to help destroy excess cells. Use 1 teaspoon herb to 1 cup boiling water and drink 1-3 cups per day.

A poultice made of burdock leaves will help to heal skin rashes and ulcerous blemishes. Change the poultice when dry and repeat as needed.

To help remove growth on any part of the body, steep 1 ounce red clover, 1 ounce burdock, 2 ounces Oregon grape leaves and ½ ounce bloodroot in 1 pint boiling water. Store in a glass container and drink 1 cup four times a day.

For minor cuts, wounds and bruises, use the beechdrops plant. Apply externally to the cut, wound or bruise to promote healing. Use in poultice form or drink in tea.

For bruises, mix the powdered root of monkshood with egg white and apply to the skin over the affected area.

A poultice of giant Solomon seal root will help to disperse congealed blood from bruises. This treatment also helps to mend broken bones. Change poultice when dry. Repeat as needed.

Powdered arnica promotes healing of cuts and bruises when sprinkled onto injured area.

Bleeding under the skin may indicate a vitamin P (hesperidin) deficiency. See the appendix for lists of foods whcih contain this vitamin.

Open wounds can be drawn together without stiches by applying comfrey poultices. Change poultices when dry and repeat as needed. Drink comfrey tea in addition to help facilitate healing.

Bunions, Corns and Calluses

Bunions, corns and calluses are most often caused by ill fitting shoes. These growths will draw fluid out of the joints and cause stiffness.

Massage corns and calluses with castor oil twice a day. The corns will peel off in layers and leave soft, smooth skin and the calluses will soften.

Boil sweet gum bark into a strong tea, cool and use daily on corns to help remove them.

For bunions, use 2 handfuls comfrey root to 1 gallon water, boil together slowly for 30 minutes, let cool and strain. Soak the feet in this tea for 10-15 minutes, both morning and night.

Apply fresh lemon juice to warts, corns and bunions daily to draw the hardened skin away. Use a lemon juice poultice during the night, changing when dry.

Warts and corns can be destroyed by external application of sun dew juice. Repeat often until the condition is cleared.

Chapped Lips and Hands
Chapped lips are an indication that the stomach is tense.

Peppermint, spearmint or camomile tea will help to soothe the stomach tension. Use 1 teaspoon herb to 1 cup boiling water and drink freely.

Rub powdered arnica onto chapped lips to soothe them. Arnica will also promote healing of wounds, bruises and irritation of the nasal passages.

Vitamin E oil and wheat germ oil will help to soothe chapped lips. Repeat application as often as needed.

For chapped hands and frost bite, rub wheat germ oil onto hands to help heal chapping and soreness.

Diaper Rash
Rub golden seal combined with lanolin onto the clean baby to help prevent urine burns and soothe rashes from diaper irritation. Repeat with each changing of the diapers.

Complexion care and Face and Skin Cleansers
Turnips are good for the complexion. Eaten daily, they will help purify the blood, reduce acidity in the system, and destroy bacteria and toxins in the body.

Dandelion greens are a good skin tonic. They help build skin cells and oxygenate the blood. Eat daily in salads or liquify in blender for a liquid tonic.

Raspberry leaf tea works internally to help clean the body internally and feed the skin. Drink 1-3 cups per day.

To soften and cleanse the face, mix ½ teaspoon egg yolk and ½ teaspoon sour cream and rub gently into the skin. Let dry for 15 minutes and wash off. For best results, repeat 2-3 times a day.

Parseley makes a good face lotion which will increase circulation and help to bring better color to the skin. This lotion also makes a good rinse for oily skin. Use 1 handful parseley in 1 pint boiling water, steep ½ hour, strain and wash the face with the mixture several times a day. Use fresh mixture each day.

For a peaches and cream complexion, use fresh peaches and cream! Mix equal parts and apply to the face. Let dry, splash with warm water and pat dry. Repeat often. Eat plenty of fresh fruits and vegetables.

Mix dried quince seeds with water using 1 teaspoon seeds to 1 pint warm or cold water. Apply 1 teaspoon liquid to the face and leave on overnight to help tighten the skin.

Brewer's yeast helps to prevent wrinkles in the face. Mix equal quantities of brewer's yeast and yogurt to make a facial. Allow to dry on the skin and splash off with warm water. Use this mixture twice a week.

Grind oak groats into a powder and make into a tea. Apply to the skin to help smoothe out wrinkles.

Aloes and camphor help to improve muscle tone in the body and are also helpful for removing wrinkles. Apply externally.

Herpes (shingles)

Herpesi is a nerve condition which may be caused by a lack of vitamins B, C, D, and sulfur. Spinach, apricots and alfalfa are helpful when treating this disease.

Mix powdered pharum phos (a cell salt) with witch hazel and apply to external eruptions. This cell salt may also be taken internally to facilitate recovery.

Add kelp to the diet to help elimiminate herpes. Use dulse, taken 1 teaspoon daily, or eat seaweed soup.

Cold Sores

Cold sores may indicate an over acidic condition in the body. Eat raw potatoes or baked potatoes without salt, butter or sour cream.

Carbuncles

Carbuncles are painful inflammations of the skin which discharge pus. A carrot or lobelia poultice applied to the affected parts helps to draw out the infection. Change the poultice often, or when dry. Repeat until the condition improves. Never open any skin eruption as this may invite further infection.

Dandruff

To fight dandruff combine ½ cup apple cider vinegar, 1 cup mint leaves and 1 cup water and boil together slowly for 5 minutes. Strain and rub the cooled mixture into the scalp. Repeat with each hair wash.

Eliminate all refined sugar and sugar products from the diet for one month and take B-complex vitamins daily to help fight dandruff.

For dandruff and alopecia (hair falling out in patches), mix 1 teaspoon bay leaf oil and 7 ounces almond oil. Paint the bald spots with the mixture daily. Continue as needed.

Eczema

☆Dandelion greens are a good treatment for eczema because they help to give oxygen to the blood and build cells. Eat in salads or drink in tea made from the root or leaves. Make the tea using 1 teaspoon herb to 1 cup boiling water and drink 1-3 cups per day.

To treat eczema, use hardboiled eggs. Cut open the egg and heat the yolk over a flame. Rub the drops from the egg yolk onto the affected areas. Repeat as often as necessary to help clear the condition.

Dab vinegar on affected areas to help control eczema. Repeat as needed.

Cucumber juice taken both internally and externally will help to clear eczema and skin eruptions. Take 1 teaspoon daily of golden seal in capsule or powder form to help clear internal causes. Golden seal tea can also be applied to the affected areas daily.

Rhatany helps to reduce the discharge from the skin and to draw tissue together. Use a poultice made of juiced rhatany leaves. Change when dry and repeat as needed.

Eating several teaspoons of watercress per day will help to control eczema and aid vision, especially night blindness.

For eczema and all skin conditions, mix ½ ounce sassafras bark, 1 ounce burdock root, 2 ounces clover and 1 pint boiling water and allow mixture to overnight. In the morning, bring to a boil and simmer for 20 minutes. Strain, and drink 2 ounces three times a day until the skin is cleared.

For dry skin, eat tree ripened figs. This fruit, added to the diet, helps to stimulate the digestive glands.

Gangrene

☆To treat gangrene, mix equal parts charcoal and whole wheat flour with enough saliva (or water) to make a paste. If possible, use the spittle from the affected person. Put this paste into a cloth and apply to affected areas. When the poultice dries, replace using a fresh cloth. Burn the used cloths. In addition, drink comfrey tea freely.

Beat fresh parkinson root into a powder and spread onto leather covered with lard. Lay the leather against gangrenous area to help bring relief. This treatment is also good for moist ulcers.

Hives

Hives can be treated by applying a mixture of cream of tartar and water. This paste should be applied often to the red marks.

Drink sassafras tea freely instead of water to help control hives. This tea helps to cleanse the blood and restore normal circulation.

Itches

☆To help stop itching and promote healing of insect bites, stings or sores, apply pure lemon juice to the affected areas. Repeat when needed. See the section on insects for further information.

To relieve itching on any part of the body, apply wheat germ oil daily. The itch should cease within two weeks.

Boil dock leaves in vinegar until soft and combine with lard to make an ointment which will help to stop itching. Apply to irritated areas when needed.

The fluid extract of grendelia (gum plant) is good for itch and ivy poisoning. Apply the juice to affected areas. Pansy and violet leaves are also effective when used this way.

Liniments for Stiff Muscles and Joints

For stiff muscles, mix 1 cup vinegar, 1 egg and 1 cup turpentine and allow the mixture to stand for 2-3 days. Rub the mixture externally into stiff joints or sore muscles.

wall flower tea is a good treatment for aches of the joints. Use 1 teaspoon to 1 cup boiling water and drink 1-3 cups daily.

To draw out stiffness from joints and muscles, use orache leaves in a poultice. Change when dry and repeat, if necessary.

Knotgrass juice, when rubbed on broken joints or ruptures, will promote healing. Repeat as necessary.

Poison Ivy, Oak and Nettles

☆ Make a tea using ¼ teaspoon golden seal to 1 cup boiling water to drink and 1 teaspoon golden seal to 1 pint water fro washing. Drink the mixture 6 times a day and wash often. About 20 minutes after the initial treatment, the itching from the poison ivy should stop.

To treat poison ivy and oak, boil 1 cup water with four cloves of chopped garlic. Let cool and apply mixture with cotton to affected parts. Repeat often. Drinking garlic tea is also helpful.

Use madrone or manzanita leaves in tea, 1 teaspoon herb to 1 cup boiling water. Drink and apply the liquid with cotton to the affected areas to help control poison ivy and oak.

For poison ivy and oak, boil jewel weed down to a mush or crush the juice from the stems of the plant and place on the affected areas. Repeat when necessary.

Crush sword fern and rub onto affected areas to help relieve pain and itching from nettle stings.

Apply wet clay to nettle stings and let dry. The clay will help to draw out the sting and reduce the swelling Repeat when dry.

Conditions of the fingers and Nails

Ring-a-round is an infection which causes the finger to swell and become painful. It will cause a ring to extend at the base of the fingernail around the finger, and indicates toxicity in the body. To relieve the swelling, use a comfrey poultice or bind a piece of fresh lemon onto the finger. Change the poultice when dry and repeat until infection is completely cleared. Fasting is also recommended to clean out the bowels and clear the system of toxins.

Alum is an effective poultice for infected or ingrown nails. Mix with enough water to make a paste and change when dry.

Ragged cuticles may indicate a calcium deficiency. Take calcium and magnesium supplements daily and eat foods which are high sources. (See appendix for lists of foods)

Psoriasis
Dap garlic oil onto the affected parts of the body with cotton to help clear up psoriasis. Repeat daily.

For psoriasis, steep 1 teaspoon sarsaparilla root in 1 cup boiling water for 15 minutes and rub onto affected areas. Repeat as often as possible.

Spots on the skin
White blotches on the arms and legs, grey hair and cold hands and feet are all indications that the body may be low in pantothenic acids. Eat only raw, natural products and eliminate all sugar and refined products from the diet.

Loss of body pigment or vitiligo may be caused by the destruction of the acid covering of the skin. Treat with pure mayonnaise which is almost totally acid. Dissolve 1 cup mayonnaise in ¼ cup boiling water with 500mg of PBA and apply to the skin on affected areas. Repeat for several days.

To help get rid of spots and blemishes on the skin, mix powdered monkshood root with egg white and apply to the skin. Repeat several times a day.

Stretch Marks
☆After a bath, smooth 1 tablespoon sesame oil over the entire body. This treatment will eventually remove stretch marks caused by weight loss, pregnancy, or scars and help to make the skin soft and young looking. Be sure to cover the entire body each time you apply the oil.

Rough, Dry, Oily, Clammy and Sweaty Skin
Rough skin may be caused by a lack of pantothenic acid in the system. This acid is found in royal jelly, honey, egg yolks, broccoli, brewer's yeast and almost all vegetables. Eat plenty of these foods daily.

Fennel tea is a good treatment for clammy skin. Use 1 teaspoon fennel to 1 cup boiling water and drink freely.

For sore, reddened hands, rub on pure lemon juice, rinse and let dry, or mix together coconut oil, olive oil and vaseline and apply to hands. Repeat several times a day.

To treat dry skin on the face, press gently as indicated in the diagram, in the order of the numbered arrows. Repeat daily. This process helps to stimulate the natural production of the facial oils.

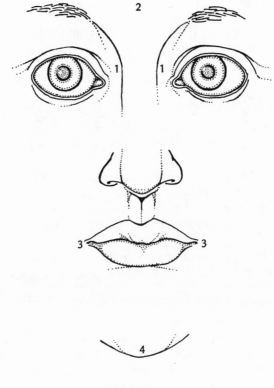

Diagram 11

Dry hands and feet usually result from gulping water and other liquids instead of sipping them. This condition may also be caused by not drinking enough liquids.

For dry, hard, scaly skin, make a tea using 1 teaspoon burdock or sunflower seeds and 1 cup boiling water. When mixture has cooled, rub into the skin several times daily until the condition clears.

For cold hands or feet, use 1 ounce prickly ash to 1 quart boiling water and steep for 15 minutes. Drink 3-4 cups per day to help stimulate the circulation and warm the body.

For sweaty feet, place the feet into water as hot as you can stand it with 1 tablespoon chlorine bleach every night and morning for about 15 minutes.

Oily skin is sometimes a result of a vitamin B_6 deficiency. This lack of B vitamins can also cause stiffness in the joints.

Running Sores
Combine black currant leaves, honeysuckle leaves, horehound and giant hyssop in equal parts and make into a tea. Apply one drop of the liquid externally to help heal running sores. Repeat daily.

Running sores on the breasts are caused by impurities of the digestive system. and blood. Use grated potatoes in a poultice on the breasts and change the poultice when dry. A cleansing diet should be initiated immediately. See the chapter on fasting for further information.

For abscesses of the breasts, use the root and leaves of the pokeroot plant in a poultice. Change the poultice when dry and repeat until abscess is drawn out.

Sagging Breasts
Take four to five tablespoons of wheat germ oil daily to help restore sagging breasts caused by nursing, weight gain or stretched muscles. Improvement should be seen within three weeks. Exercises should be taken in conjunction to help strengthen the chest muscles.

Styes

Styes may indicate that the liver is congested. Collect your own urine from the first elimination in the morning and dab onto the sty to help reduce it. Also use the cleansing diet recommended in the liver section.

Swelling

☆ Use watercress, comfrey or crushed ivy in poultice form to relieve swelling anywhere in the body.

Warts

Warts on the body may indicate that there is excess lime in the system, and that body resistance to infection is low. Camomile tea helps to neutralize the excess lime and should be taken 2-3 times per day. Here are some other methods of treating warts.

For warts on the genitals, use the outside skin of the pineapple and rub onto the affected parts. Repeat morning and evening until the warts are gone.

Apply milkweed "milk" to warts daily to help destroy them.

The inside milk from unripe red figs will help get rid of warts. Apply externally once or twice a day until cleared.

To remove warts, use the spittle from the mouth taken first thing in the morning and dab onto the wart. Repeat daily until the warts disappear.

☆Apply vitamin E or wheat germ oil to warts daily to help remove them.

Sun dew juice applied externally will help to destroy warts and corns.

House leek leaves contain malt that helps to remove warts. Chop the leaves and use 1 teaspoon leaves to 1 cup boiling water. Drink 1 cup per day and apply cooled mixture externally to warts.

Soaking the hands in cooled water which eggs have been boiled in will help to get rid of warts on the hands.

Miscellaneous

Leprosy can be treated with calamint. Use about 1 teaspoon to 1 cup boiling water, steep several minutes and strain. Apply externally to the skin and drink several cups per day. Repeat applications often.

Bumps on the fingers can be caused by eating different kinds of fruits at the same time. The combinations of acids in the fruit cause the bumps. Eat only one kind of fruit per day.

Thyroid dysfunctions can cause skin disorders. Take dulse (ground sea weed) daily to treat this condition. Massage the corresponding area of the feet as illustrated in the Feet and Legs section diagram to stimulate the thyroid.

TEETH AND GUMS

Your teeth should last a lifetime and if cared for properly, they will remain strong and healthy. Teeth respond to vitamin C and need calcium long after their formative years. Toothaches and abscesses are a signal that there is an obstruction somewhere in the digestive system and a cleansing diet is recommended. Sometimes the obstruction is due to mucous which will not be blocking the system but may be inhibiting digestion.

Decay Prevention
Strawberries cut in half and rubbed into the teeth and gums help to remove tartar on the teeth and to strengthen and heal gums. Leave the juice on for as long as possible (up to 45 min) then rinse the mouth with warm water. Use only fresh strawberries.

Lemon juice and rind help to remove plaque and tartar on the teeth when mixed with the saliva in the mouth. "Chew" the juice to make sure it is throughly mixed with saliva then swallow slowly. Repeat at least once a week. Scrub the teeth with lemon rind and make sure all surfaces are treated. The upper gums should be massaged down and the lower gums massaged up. Lime juice or rind may be used instead as both kill bacteria in the mouth when used with warm water.

Alfalfa tablets help to prevent dental cavities. Take two tablets 2-3 times per day.

Lemon juice and flower pumice mixed together should be used once a month to remove any tartar deposits on the teeth.

Parseley tonic helps strengthen the teeth. Use 1 quart boiling water poured over 1 cup packed parsley. Steep 15 minutes and strain. Refrigerate the mixture and drink 3 cups per day.

Barley is excellent for all diseases of the teeth and gums. Use in soups or stews.

Witch hazel is a good mouthwash but should not be swallowed.

The powdered root of water dock is valuable for cleansing the mouth. Use 1 ounce powdered herb to 1 pint boiling water and steep for 5 minutes. Rinse mouth two times a day.

Powdered dock is a good dentifrice and may be used instead of toothpaste.

Red sage is a cleansing gargle. Mix 1 pint malt vinegar, 1 ounce red sage leaves, and ½ pint cold water. Gargle ½ cup two times a day.

Toothaches
Aloe vera helps soothe toothache pain. Use juice of plant on gums and repeat often.

Cloves help remove toothache pain and may be used in many ways. The oil can be rubbed into the gums, whole cloves may be sucked for their juices, or the cloves may be mixed with boiling water to make a tea or gargle.

Chewing prickly ash bark helps to relieve toothache pain.

Mullein flowers when used in a poultice help to draw out the pain of toothache. Use flowers and warm water, strain and use the moist flowers in poultice form on the outside of the mouth.

Egg yolk and honey, mixed together and placed on the skin outside the jaw, help draw out pain from wisdom teeth.

Milk from ripe figs is good for toothaches. Squeeze out the juice and rub onto gums around tooth.

☆Gentle pressure applied to the sides of the index finger on either hand helps relieve toothache pains and relax the tension caused by pain (see diagram 12).

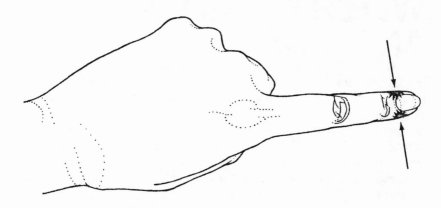

To help relieve toothache pain, apply pressure as indicated.

Diagram 12

Trench Mouth, Thrush and Mouth Ulcers
A mixture of golden seal and myrrh is excellent for trench mouth. Use equal parts of each and massage gums (upper gums down and lower gums up). Also use with warm water to gargle. This mixture works well for bleeding gums also.

Acacia bark is useful for ulcers of the mouth and gums, and to help secure loose teeth. Use ½ teaspoon in 1 cup boiling water and gargle several times per day.

Arsesmart leaves help to heal ulcers in the mouth. Use 1 ounce leaves to 1 pint boiling water. Drink 1 pint or more of the mixture per day, 3 ounces at a time.

Baby Teething
☆Rubbing the gums with olive oil helps relieve soreness and lubricate the digestive system.

Teething babies can be helped through this painful period with camomile tea. Use ½ teaspoon camomile to 1 cup boiling water. Steep 3-4 minutes, strain and sweeten with honey. Test for temperature and give the baby 2-3 teaspoons several times a day as needed.

WEIGHT GAIN AND LOSS

Millions of Americans are overweight. As we are affluent, so are we over-fed. Carrying around excess pounds puts a strain on the heart and on the digestive system. Before embarking on a weight loss program, you should check to be sure that the problem is not due to a thyroid condition or other organ malfunction. If it is, then you must work to restore that organ to proper functioning before attempting to lose the weight it has caused you to gain. Once you have ascertained that all the organs are functioning properly you must examine and correct your diet, exercise program and mental attitude towards weight loss.

To lose weight, you should eat only non glue foods, and eat only when you are hungry. Each person's eating schedule will be unique, so plan your meals according to your stomach and not according to the clock. Avoid processed foods as they are high in calories and low in nutritive values.

The best diet in the world will not help much if you do not get proper exercise. Plan an exercise program for yourself which will give you the needed movement, but do not plan an elaborate program which will not fit in your schedule and which you will be tempted to drop after one week. Walking one extra mile per day will help to take off one pound per week! Proper exercise will stimulate the system to eliminate wastes and burn off excess fat. Raw fruits and vegetables and high protein meats such as fish, poultry and lean red meats will provide energy without putting on fat. Lecithin, a derivative of the soybean, will help to break down fatty cholesterol deposits. Lecithin contains phosphorus and 1-2 tablespoons per day will help to stimulate the metabolism.

Make up your mind that you are getting slimmer every day. Thinking about the weight that you will gain while eating a hot fudge sundae will only make you feel heavier and depressed, and more likely to eat more. The mind controls how you feel about your body and can help you lose weight without changing much of your diet at all. Deciding to lose weight is the key. I have personally found that I can lose four or five pounds within a week if I make up my mind to do so. On the other hand, if you do not believe that you have "will power" to lose weight, you are mentally preparing yourself not to do so.

Weight Loss

The following foods are glue foods, and should be avoided if you intend to lose weight. These foods interfere with the pituitary gland and hinder the ability of the hormones to metabolize fats. Glue foods literally stick to your intestinal tract and promote weight gain:

white flour	white sugar
sweet potatoes	ice cream
all bakery products	bread
soft drinks	crackers
french toast	potato chips
frozen creamed vegetables	ale
candy	canned fruit
sweet wines	biscuits
yams	processed cereal
waffles	pancakes
pasta	doughnuts
jam	beer

The following foods are easier to digest and help to support the energy needs of the body without adding fat:

whole grain cereals	rice flour
steamed vegetables	lettuce
brown rice	raw vegetables
alfalfa sprouts	all bean sprouts
grapefruit	all seafood
all fresh fruits	gelatin
sea plants	turkey
all vegetable juices	chicken

Here are some aids to weight loss:

Before a meal, mash two bananas throughly and combine with 8 ounces soy or goat milk. Skim milk may be used if soy or goat milk is unavailable. Blend together and drink slowly 1 hour before the meal. At mealtime your appetite will be reduced considerably. Two glasses of this mixture can be used to replace the meal.

Two ounces of grapefruit juice mixed with 1 ounce plain water and sipped slowly ½ to 1 hour before a meal will help to prevent the body from taking on weight.

Cleaver's herb stimulates weight loss. Make the leaves into a tea using 1 ounce to 1 quart boiling water. Drink three or more cups per day. For the first six weeks, very little effect will be noticed but beginning with the seventh week of treatment, the effects will become noticeable. Cleaver's herb helps the body to metabolize and throw off fatty substances through the urine. To maximize the effects of cleaver's herb, combine with fennel or seaweed.

Steam chickweed greens and mix with wild mustard, shepherd's purse, or peppergrass to help weight loss. Eat the chickweed mixture and drink the broth.

Bamboo shoots are helpful in losing excess weight. Eat the tender shoots raw, or soften by boiling for 5-10 minutes.

Yerba mate helps decrease the sensation of hunger and aids digestion while supplying vitamin C to the body. Use 1 teaspoon to 1 cup boiling water. Drink 4 cups per day.

The inner bark of white ash is effective for weight loss. Steep a heaping teaspoon in 1 cup boiling water for ½ hour. Drink 4 ounces daily.

Weight Gain

To gain weight, do not eat "fattening" foods as they will only put a strain on the body. Eat instead good, nourishing foods and foods high in B-complex vitamins to help stimulate the appetite and nourish the system. Barley contains large amounts of B vitamins and should be eaten daily in soups, stews, or other cooked foods.

To improve the appetite steep together ½ cup clover and ½ cup boiling water. Add ½ teaspoon lemon juice and strain and take 1 tablespoon 3-6 times a day.

Boil 1 handful dogwood bark in 1 quart water down to 1 pint. Let the mixture stand for 1 hour. Strain and take 1 tablespoon three times a day before meals.

Tightly pack 1 teaspoon each wild cherry bark, red alder bark and cedar bark in a container and cover with boiling water. Take up to 5 cups per day of this mixture including one just before bedtime.

WORMS

Almost everyone will have worms at some point in their life. They can easily be picked up from the soil, from foods and from pets, but getting rid of worms is not very difficult. There are three main ways of checking for worms. Observe your eating habits. If you do have worms, you will tend to eat far more than usual, and feel hungry more frequently. Check the feces for worms, but this is not a positive test as some are very difficult to see. while other may be external rather than in the digestive tract. Check the base of the nose. If worms are in the system, there will be a small line extending outward towards the ears on either side of the nostrils. Some worms, such as ringworm, will produce a "ring" on the skin. Usually this ring will appear near the elbow or knee, but worms will lodge anywhere in the body that is warm and moist.

All Worms
☆Garlic is the most effective remedy for worms of all types. First thing in the morning, chop one clove of garlic and place in a spoon. Fill the spoon the rest of the way with olive or sesame oil and swallow. Do not eat or drink anything until the bowels have moved. Repeat the next day and check feces. If necessary, repeat the third day.

Mix ½ ounce each of tansy, wormwood and camomile with 1 pint boiling water. Steep for five minutes. Drink ½ cup and wait two hours before eating or drinking anything.

The fruit of the wormwood tree helps to expel worms. Mix 2 ounces of the bark or 20 grains of the pulp with 1 pint boiling water. Boil the mixture down to ½ pint and take 1 tablespoon 1-3 hours before bedtime. Repeat two times the first week, once the second week and thereafter once a month to remain free of worms.

Eat young, tender bamboo shoots boiled in water for 10 minutes to help expel worms. Eat the shoots twice a day for 1 week.

Pomegranates contain a substance which kills worms in the intestinal tract.

The skin of the tree root is the most powerful part. Use ½ teaspoon pomegranate tree root skin to 1 cup boiling water and steep for 15 minutes. Drink ½ cup twice a day for three days.

The papain from papaya seeds is effective for expelling worms. Eat 1 tablespoon or drink 1 cup tea made from the seeds each day.

Crushed green walnut hulls made into a tea are a good remedy for ringworm and tapeworm. Use ½ teaspoon hulls to 1 cup boiling water. Drink 2 cups per day.

To rid the body of tapeworms, follow this diet for eight days. Every waking hour, drink 1 cup of tea made from 2 tablespoons each of crushed pomegranates and crushed male fern root to 1 quart boiling water. Starting with the second day, take a tablespoon of castor oil with each cup of tea. In addition, eat 1 handful of pumpkin seeds every three hours. During this eight day fast, you may sip beef or chicken broth if you are hungry.

CHAPTER 4

EMERGENCY PROCEDURES

EMERGENCY PROCEDURES

True emergency situations are rare, but being prepared can turn a nightmare into a momentary discomfort. Shock is the most common emergency problem, occurring whenever there is a major mental, physical or emotional disturbance in the system. In shock, the body produces excess adrenalin to offset the emergency and provide energy for escape. This is a defense mechanism, and has provided the energy for people to lift cars from on top of loved ones or run at incredible speeds in order to save their lives. Without this kind of physical exertion, the body must find other ways to eliminate the excess adrenalin and restore normal functioning. Have the patient breathe fresh, clean air. If you are inside stand or seat the patient in front of an open window. Massage the feet around the areas corresponding to the pancreas and the organs or part of the body affected by the shock. See the Feet and Legs section for diagrams 6 and 7. The wrist snap, diagram 13, will stimulate the heart and circulatory system to promote elimination of the excess adrenalin.

Edward Bach, a British naturalist, mixed together the herbs Star of Bethlehem, Rock Rose, Impatiens, Cherry Plum, and Clematis to make what he calls "Rescue Remedy". This mixture can be ordered from England (see the appendix for the address) and is specifically used for treating shock. Add 1 drop of the concentrated mixture to 1 ounce water and at intervals of 15 minutes to 30 minutes, place a small amount on the tongue. After 1 hour reduce the frequency of usage. The amount will vary from patient to patient and according to the severity of the shock. When dealing with shock victims, this remedy is nice to have on hand to help until further assistance can arrive and to give comfort to the patient.

Cortisone
Cortisone treatments create severe deficiencies in the body. Prolonged cortisone treatments may cause softening of the bones and make them break easily. Dessicated liver, bone meal, vitamin C and alfalfa tablets should be taken daily during the treatment and for several weeks after it has been discontinued. It is recommended that you avoid cortisone entirely. Alternatives to cortisone treatments are listed in the sections dealing with specific diseases.

Trick Knees
To treat trick knees and popping joints, take bone meal and dolomite. To replace an out-of-place knee, kneel on the other leg, and stand slowly. As you stand, the kneecap will be freed and will slip into correct position. This pro-

cess may be repeated several times. A poultice of comfrey leaves or tea may be used on the knee to insure proper repair. Make comfrey tea, using 1 teaspoon leaves to 1 cup boiling water, and drink 4-5 cups per day for 3 days, then 1-3 cups per day for several weeks.

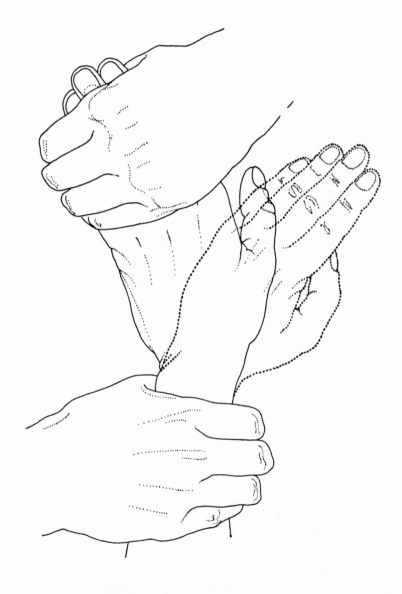

Diagram 13 Wrist snap treatment for shock

Bleeding and Hemorrhaging

To stop excessive bleeding, make a tea of shepherd's purse. This tea contains large quantities of vitamins C and K which help the blood to clot, sometimes within 15 minutes. Use 1 teaspoon shepherd's purse leaves to 1 cup boiling water, steep for 3-5 minutes and sip the warm tea slowly. Take 1-3 cups daily or as needed.

Vitamin C and vitamin P (Hesperidin) will help to stop hemorrhages. Take up to 500 mg. per day.

To stop bleeding, gently press both legs on the inside of the leg, 5 inches below the knee. Hold this pressure for several minutes or until bleeding stops. (See diagram 14).

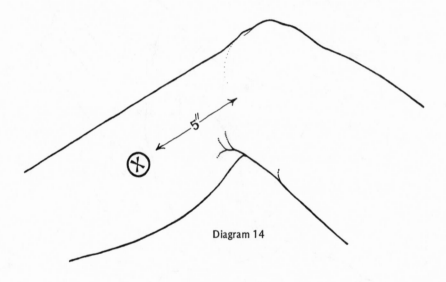

Diagram 14

Food Poisoning

Drink ½ cup olive oil slowly to help facilitate removal of the poison in the system. Repeat six hours later, if necessary.

Take ½ glass hot water with 1 teaspoon baking soda in it to help relax and calm the system and remove the poison food.

Arsenic Poisoning

Ingested arsenic will settle in the eyes and back muscles and may cause muscle spasms, paralysis or softening of the bones. Take teas of herbs that contain sulfur, such as nettle, dock, fennel or bullweed. Use 1 teaspoon of any of these herbs in 1 cup boiling water, steep for 3-5 minutes and drink 3 cups per day. Begin a raw vegetable juice diet of carrot, spinach, celery, parseley and beet juices to help cleanse the system.

Scorpion, Snake, Spider and Insect Bites
Rue is an antidote for scorpion, snake, spider and insect poisoning Make a tea of rue leaves using 1 teaspoon to 1 cup boiling water, steep 5 minutes, Strain and drink 2-3 cups as necessary. The strained leaves may be used as a poultice on the affected area.

Radiation Poisoning
Mix 1 teaspoon baking soda, 1 teaspoon salt, and 1 quart water and drink 18 ounces every 2 hours, if the condition is severe. When the symptoms appear in the head, chest, throat, glandular system or nasal cavity add ½ teaspoon cream of tartar to the solution. Continue treatment until all symptoms are gone. With each glass of the liquid take 3-5 grains of calcium.

Smoke Inhalation
Use flaxseed tea to treat excessive smoke inhalation from burning buildings, tear gas, etc. Use 1 teaspoon flaxseed to 1 pint water, bring the mixture to a boil, and steep for 5-10 minutes. Strain and sip slowly. Honey may be used as a sweetener if necessary as it also helps to soothe the membranes of the throat.

Slippery elm bark is also a good treatment for smoke inhalation. Make the powdered bark into a tea or mix with warm water and honey to make a gargle.

Whiplash
Whiplash results when the neck is subjected to sudden shock or movement which the muscles are too tense to absorb. Neck collars are the worst treatment you can use for whiplash! They do not help the neck to re-align nor do they give the body a chance to help itself work back into place. See a Naturopath, Osteopath or Chiropractor and have the neck vertebrae realigned. Place a silk scarf or cloth on the neck and wear it. The silk keeps the blood moving and helps to relieve pain and tension in the muscles.

To Avoid Contagious Disease

Hold juniper berries under the tongue to protect yourself from contagious diseases. They may be changed when soggy, and the berries help to prevent infection from entering the body.

Make dittany into a tea and rub onto the body to help protect against contagion.

Alfalfa tea, taken daily, will help to build up the body resistance to disease. The tablets may be used instead of the tea.

Cramps

Raspberry tea will help to soothe cramping muscles. Use 1 ounce leaves in 1 pint water and simmer for 20 minutes. Drink the liquid and use the pulp as a poultice on the affected area.

Hiccups

Dill leaf tea will help to stop hiccups. Use 1 teaspoon dill to 1 cup boiling water. Sip slowly to help equalize the oxygen in the bloodstream and diaphragm.

Sprains, Fractures and Broken Bones

Comfrey (also called knitbone) helps to reduce swelling of sprains, and to draw fractured bone fragments back together. Use a poultice of fresh leaves, apply to the affected area . The poultices should be changed several times per day. If fresh comfrey is not available, the dried leaves may be used. In addition, use one teaspoon comfrey leaves to one cup boiling water and drink 2-3 cups per day. The tea will help facilitate healing.

CHAPTER 5

FASTING

FASTING

Fasting is an old custom, originating in ancient ritual, designed to promote health. The purpose of a fast is to cleanse the system of undigested residue, to stimulate the organs and glands, and to revitalize the entire system. Fasting does not necessarily mean abstaining from food, but does entail following a specific diet of foods, liquids or a combination of both. Fasting should never result in dizziness, nausea or fatigue.

Many popular fasts may be detrimental to your health. A fast consisting of only water is valuable only in specific instances and not for prolonged periods of time. Water contains little nourishment and cannot cleanse the glandular system effectively or expel mucous from the digestive tract. Fasting for the first 10 hours of the day and then eating a heavy meal will drastically alter the metabolism and shock the system. It is not effective to try to combine eating with fasting. A fast should be followed for at least 24 hours or should not be attempted. Repeated fasting for one or more days a week, for months on end, will cause the stomach to repeatedly shrink and expand and may eventually harm the natural elasticity of the organ. Fasting for extreme periods of time may deplete vitamin and mineral reserves so badly that the body must metabolize its own bone marrow in order to continue functioning.

If you are mentally and physically prepared, however, fasting can be very beneficial to your health. A fast during an illness, such as a strict juice fast during a cold, can help the system to fight infection and heal wounds. In fact, many of the treatments in this book are fasts.

The length of a fast should be determined by your schedule. Do not attempt to fast when you are particularly busy or under severe mental or physical stress. It is important to remember that your method of ending a fast is just as vital as your method of fasting. At the end of this chapter, I have included some thoughts which will help you to break a fast without discomfort and without destroying the benefits of the fast.

General Fast

☆This fast is cleansing for the entire system. Combine 6 ounces papaya concentrate, 4 ounces prune juice, 4 ounces fresh pinapple juice, 8 ounces orange juice with 1 quart distilled water. Set aside a second quart of distilled water. Once an hour, or less often if you do not feel thirsty, drink 4 ounces of the mixture and 4 ounces of the distilled water from the second quart. You may use this fast for from 1 days to 1 month. A three day fast will cleanse the entire body. This is the only fast I have been able to use without experiencing hunger pains. If you are unused to fasting, this is one of the most pleasant. Be sure all the ingredients are organic and the distilled water is pure. Tap water which has been chlorinated will inhibit the benefits of the fast.

Rice and Fish Fast

A 10 day diet of nothing but fish and brown rice will cleanse the entire system, rejuvenate the spleen and re-mineralize a sluggish body. Use short grain organic brown rice as it is the most nutricious. You may eat any type of fish and you should try to eat a variety of fish over the 10 days.

Two Day Cleansing Diet

For two days, eat nothing but raw vegetables of all kinds and sip three eight ounce glasses of distilled water per day. Do not eat or drink anything else. This fast will rid the body of debris in the system and help metabolize the carbohydrates already present. In addition, the fast will stimulate digestive enzymes and tone the intestinal tract.

How to Break A Fast

How you stop your fast is very important. The stomach is smaller and the body is clean. If you immediately help yourself to a steak or pizza, you will shock the entire system and destroy the benefits of your days of fasting. Do not immediately eat something that will be hard to digest, or you will probably get sick. Here is a sample diet for breaking a fast.

On day one, eat an apple and sip slowly a small bowl of fresh vegetable broth or soup. Do not use any salt or spice.

On day two, repeat the menu for day one, adding a small portion of mashed potatoes, a glass of sour milk or some yogurt.

On day three, increase the portions of the above foods, adding a small amount of raw vegetable salad, a small portion of brown rice, and some fresh cottage cheese.

On day four, start to eat normally. Between meal snacks should consist of fruit only.

During the four day diet, be sure to continue drinking plenty of water and fresh juices.

CHAPTER 6

PLANTS
&
PETS

PLANTS AND PETS

Most of the remedies recommended for people will also help your animals. Domestic animals such as dogs and cats usually need more variety and nutrients than is found in their food. Herbs and supplemental vitamins may be added to food and drinking water to help restore health.

Dehydration

Dehydration constitutes a major emergency for cats and may be lethal if not treated immediately. To check for dehydration, pull the scruff of the neck of the animal. If the skin is slow in moving back into place your animal is dehydrated. Check immediately for diarrhea and make a pot of comfrey tea. Use 1 teaspoon comfrey to 1 cup boiling water and steep for 5-10 minutes. If the animal will not drink, force feed approximately 1-2 ounces of the cooled tea per hour depending on body weight. Cats, especially, get depressed if they don't feel well and will curl up and die if they are not given plenty of love and attention. The most common causes of dehydration are worms, intestinal viruses and obstructions of the intestinal tract.

Kelp is a highly nutricious food which will help to stimulate the animal's system. Soak a little kelp in water overnight. In the morning, add 1 tablespoon to the drinking water. Freshly cooked vegetables, especially carrots, celery or peas, may be added to the animal's food.

Diarrhea

Diarrhea, in animals and people, indicates that the body is throwing off poisons from the system. Diarrhea is very dangerous to animals and should be treated promptly and with a great deal of care. Veterinarians can sometimes give intravenous injections of a balanced nutritional supplement which can help to restore proper functioning of the system. Diarrhea in cats, especially kittens, may be caused by too rich foods, such as horse meat, or by eating too much too quickly.

To treat diarrhea give 1 teaspoon carob powder in 1 glass water morning and evening. If the condition is severe, force feed ½-1 glass every two hours. This amount varies according to the size of the animal.

Vitamin B helps to restore balance to the upset system. Give brewer's yeast powder or mix with meals to help rebalance the bacteria in the system.

Yogurt helps to replace and restore intestinal bacteria in all infections of the digestive tract.

Conjunctivitis
Conjunctivitis can be treated with goat milk or goat milk yogurt. Give the animal ½ - ¾ cup per day. Supplemental vitamins can also help this condition, especially vitamin A.

Eczema
To treat eczema on animals, combine 2 tablespoons cottage cheese, 2 tablespoons corn oil, 1 teaspoon wheat germ oil and 1 garlic pearly and rub onto affected area. Repeat at least once a day. Check the diet carefully as this condition usually indicates some congestion in the digestive tract.

Mange
To treat mange, mix equal parts of tar and bacon grease and apply to affected parts. Repeat 2-3 times per day until condition clears. Give B-complex vitamins or brewer's yeast tablets daily to help facilitate healing.

Gas
Many animals, especially kittens, are plagued with gas. This is usually caused by unfamiliar foods in the system which are not as readily assimilated as is mother's milk. For gas, comfrey tea is helpful when added to the food or the water bowl. Massaging the paws also helps to relieve gas pains. The Feet and Legs section of the Remedies chapter contains a diagram of the human foot whichcan be used as a guide.

Fever
Animals run a fever when the body poisons are not being thrown off properly as this is nature's way of preventing toxemia. Give a strong mixture of comfrey tea to help bring down the fever quickly and restore balance to the system. Use 1 teaspoon comfrey leaves or root and 1 cup boiling water. Steep for 10-15 minutes, and force feed, if necessary, 3-5 ounces per day. The dosage depends upon the size of the animal. For kittens use 2-3 ounces and for large dogs 5 or more ounces. Comfrey tea added to the drinking water will also help to build up resistance to disease.

Animal Cancer and External Growths
Vitamins E and A help to protect animals against cancer of the lungs and internal organs. Start by adding small dosages to foods and gradually increase up to 200 i.u. daily. These vitamins will help the animal's system to be more able to control excess cell growth.

Give garlic pearlies four times a day to help animals throw off cancer. The garlic also keeps the system clean which aids in restoring balances of vitamins and minerals. A vitamin supplement is recommended and plenty of fresh water.

Intestinal Infections (Viruses)
Yogurt, especially goat milk yogurt, helps to restore the natural bacterial balance in the animal's system and replenish diseased cells. Yogurt is especially important if the animal has been given antibiotics. These drugs destroy beneficial bacteria and the yogurt helps to replace natural intestinal enzymes.

Pregnancy
Animals, like people, need extra nutrition during pregnancy. Vitamins B,C, and E should be included in the diet as well as rolled oats and cottage cheese several times a week.

Raspberry tea should be given instead of regular drinking water to help insure an easy birth. Make a tea using 1 teaspoon raspberry leaves to 1 cup boiling water, steep for 5 minutes and add to fresh drinking water daily. This tea also supplies many vitamins and minerals.

After Birthing Needs
Pennyroyal will help to draw the female organs back into place after birth. Use 1 teaspoon herb to 1 cup boiling water and give instead of or combined with drinking water for 5-10 days.

Animal Jaundice
For animal jaundice give only water and 4 garlic pearlies per day. Do not feed as feeding puts more strain on the already overtaxed liver and prolongs the jaundice. Continue for 3-4 days.

Fleas, Ticks and Bugs
Animal flea collars are filled with a nerve gas and DDT. If wet, broken or otherwise altered, and sometimes without alteration, these gasses can cause extreme reactions in the animals. Flea collars have been known to cause all the hair around the neck to fall out, to create eye infections, and to cause severe skin burns, and even death. If you have a flea collar on your pet, or are thinking about buying one, check carefully for any unusual reactions and remove it immediately if they occur.

A pillow stuffed with pennyroyal, camomile, eucalyptus, winter savory, rosemary or mint, or a combination of these herbs will help to drive fleas away from your pet or its bed. Use in the regular sleeping place of the animal.

Rub rosemary oil into your animals' brush before grooming. This will help to drive the fleas away and leave a nice scent. Use daily during the flea season.

Make a collar of leather or cloth soaked in pennyroyal oil or eucalyptus oil, String with fresh eucalyptus buttons to keep fleas off pets.

Lockjaw
Lockjaw can be caused by infections from unclean utensils, bacterial filled horn cuts which are capped off or from a goat deciding to scratch the "itch" where his horns used to be. This disease can cause severe illness and death if not treated. The best way to insure that the toxins will be drawn out is to apply a poultice of tobacco. Make a paste of water and pure tobacco. Put this mixture in the poultice and bind in place. Change the poultice several times a day and continue until at least 2 days after the infection is gone and health is restored. The poultice cloth should be burned after use and replaced with a new cloth. Do not use cigarette tobacco as it may contain chemical impurities.

Give garlic daily in conjunction with the tobacco treatment to help keep the system clean and destroy harmful internal bacteria.

Animal Arthritis
Animal arthritis is caused by an over acid condition of the system. Vitamin B is essential for treatment, and meat consumption should be reduced and supplemented with comfrey tea and flaxseed tea as well as natural foods and grains. Use 1 teaspoon each of comfrey and flaxseed to 1 cup boiling water and steep for 10 minutes, cool, and feed to the animal. This tea may be used instead of pure water if the condition is a chronic one. There are other treatments in the Arthritis section of the Remedies Chapter that can be adapted to animal use.

Plants
Most plants need specific treatments dependent upon their variety. This section is meant only as a general informational section to deal with common problems.

Bugs, Moths and Insect Pests
Soak 5-15 juniper berries overnight in 2 cups water. In the morning, strain the mixture, add 1 quart fresh water to the liquid and spray onto plants. Repeat after rains or when needed. This spray may be used indoors or out on all kinds of herbs, flowers and vegetables. Rose bushes are expecially happy if sprayed with juniper water. The soaked berries may be dropped around the

base of the plants to protect the plant at ground level.

Use tobacco water, fixed the same as the preceeding remedy, to prevent bugs from infesting plants.

Spread coffee grounds, sassafras, or even cigarette ashes around plants to keep crawling bugs from them.

A simple collar of paper placed on the ground around the root of vegetable plants such as tomato plants will prevent cut worms from killing them.

Puny, Drooping Plants
Castor oil or cod liver oil is a good way to make your unhappy plants perk up again. Just put ½ teaspoon on the earth around the bottom of the stalk. The castor oil sinks into the soil and feeds the roots of the plants. This treatment usually produces results within several hours.

APPENDICES

ELEMENTS AND MINERALS	USE	SOURCE
CALCIUM	builds bones, teeth and aids clotting of the blood. Helps to prevent hemorrhaging and inflammation and insure normal muscle and nerve response.	asparagus, beans, cauliflower, clams, beets cabbage, carrots, celery, goat milk, goat cheese, almonds, onions, greens, lemons, tangerines, elderberries, nettle, watercress, turnips, turnip tops, alfalfa, horsetail herb, kohlrabi, raspberry leaves and pumpkin seeds.
CARBON	helps build strong bones and stimulates the body heat.	all types of fish, meats and eggs.
CHLORINE	necessary for normal digestion. Helps activate gastric secretions and enzymes.	cheese, cabbage, celery, dates, eggs, endive, fish, potatoes, oysters, spinach, onions and sauerkraut.
COBALT	controls the regulation of the appetite.	liver, seafood, leafy vegetables, whole cereals, beans of all types, apples, gelatin and onions.
COPPER	necessary for the formation of iron and hemo-globin.	beans, liver, mushrooms, peas, leafy vegetables, nuts, seafood, red and black currants;, whole grains, kale, potatoes, asparagus, peaches, bran and watercress.
FLORINE	protects and preserves the bones.	red wheat, beets, dairy products, cabbage, garlic, spinach, seafoods, whole wheat, rye, and watercress.
HYDROGEN	necessary for elimination, perspiration and the salivary processes as well as the growth of blood cells and the circulation of the blood. Helps to soothe the nerves and regulate the body temperature.	lemons, oranges, limes, grapes, peaches, plums, cherries, tomatoes, grapefruit, fresh pineapple and watermelon.

IODINE	necessary for thyroid health and gland functions. Needed for normal metabolism.	seafood of all kinds, sea plants, bran, broccoli, butter, carrots, spinach, cherries, onions, garlic, figs, mushrooms, oats, almonds, asparagus, beans, kale, celery , chard, dandelion, egg yolks, kidney, hearts, liver, currents, prunes, dates, raisons, watercress, oranges, and poultry.
IRON	necessary for the development of red corpuscles and to carry oxygen to the cells.	almonds, honey, coconuts, beets, beet greens, kale, cauliflower, celery, dandelion, chard, egg yolks, hearts, kidneys, liver, seafood of all types, dates, prunes, raisins, watercress, oranges, poultry, red and black currents, raspberries and raspberry leaves, apricots, parsley, nettles, alfalfa, red clover blossoms, baked beans, kidney beans, rolled oats, red poppy, caraway, anise, rosemary, fennel, sage, calendula and pumpkin seeds.
LIME	aids digestion in the stomach.	coconuts, limes, cottage cheese and soy beans.
MAGNESIUM	influences the muscles, essential to the bone structure and the nerves. Activates enzymes needed for digestive processes.	honey, almonds, barley, chard, cress, beans, clams, corn, peas, prunes, figs, lraisins; potatoes, dates, parsnips, green cabbage, dandelion, brussel sprouts, bananas, carrots, fish, elderberries, lemons, raspberries, endive, nettle, alfalfa and watercress.

ELEMENTS AND MINERALS	USE	SOURCE
MANGANESE	essential for growth and to aid tissue respiration.	bananas, beans, beets, bran, chard, peas, leafy vegetables of all types, whole grains and almonds.
NICKEL	aids the assimilation of sugars in the system.	bean sprouts, lettuce, green beans, onions, garlic, all sea plants, shell fish, radishes, celery, tomatoes and all fresh greens.
NITROGEN	builds muscle tone, repairs and builds muscle tissues.	beans, dairy products, shellfish, nuts, lentils, wheat germ, crab, lobster, salmon and oatmeal.
OXYGEN	necessary to dissolve waste products and stimulate circulation. Feeds and stimulates all the body organs.	all fruits and vegetables with apples containing the highest amounts.
PANTOTHENIC ACID	essential for the healthy functioning of all the organs.	honey, peanuts, broccoli and all fresh vegetable juices.
PHOSPHORUS	combines with calcium to help build the bones, helps to keep the system alkaline, activate enzymes and metabolism of fatty foods and carbohydrates.	apples, alfalfa, almonds, barley, beans, bran, cheese, eggs, lentils, liver, milk, asparagus, cabbage, corn, celery, cauliflower, fish, figs, rye, whole wheat, peas, lettuce, spinach, tomatoes, grapes, raspberries, tangerines, watercress, kale, lecithin and all soy products, sweet flag, chickweed, caraway, horsetail herb, apple seeds, and pumpkin seeds.

POTASSIUM	essential to normal growth, healthy muscles, and the nerves.	alfalfa, beans, olives, bran, parsnips, pomegranates, nuts, prunes, potatoes, celery, raisins, spinach, cherries, lettuce, lemons, kale, green leafy vegetables of all kinds, bananas, beets, cabbage, carrots, grapes and tangerines.
SODIUM	protects the tissues when water is lost from the body.	kelp, tomatoes, dandelion, peaches, cheese, clams, oysters, beef, beets, olives, raisins, carrots, milk, chard, turnips, cress, wheat germ, celery, eggs, spinach and cherries.
SILICON and SELENIUM	necessary for healthy hair, skin, nails, and an aid to the mucous membranes and blood vessels. Useful in exhaustion, impotency and general mineral deficiencies.	okra, onions, oatstraw, horsetail herb, barley, brewer's yeast, oats, wheat germ and sesame oil.
SULFUR	necessary for assimilation of body protein, important for the liver and skin cells and for the entire metabolism.	beans, bullweed, nettles, cheese, eggs, nuts, bran, fish, lean meats, chard, onions, turnips, cauliflower, black and red currents, oysters, leeks, spinach, kale, coltsfoot, eyebright and fennel.
ZINC	necessary for normal growth, nerves and healthy functioning of the heart.	oysters, beets, broccoli, wheat germ, wheat bran, milk, egg yolks, peas, beans, cress, liver, dandelion, lentils, seeds, spinach, fish, red lettuce, apples, cabbage and nuts.

VITAMIN	USE	SOURCE
VITAMIN A	aids vision, promotes growth and prevents infection.	wheat, Jerusalem artichokes, parseley, string beans, green peppers, liver, eggs, butter, cream, whole milk, cheese, red salmon, tomatoes, olives, green and yellow vegetables and fruits.
VITAMIN B_1	the entire B-complex improves appetite, tones the muscles, helps prevent nervous disorders, helps stop muscle cramping and acts as a general stimulant to the system.	bell peppers, sunflower seeds, prunes, peaches, artichokes, string beans, barley, spinach, dandelion and rosehips.
VITAMIN B_2	riboflavin is essential to children's growth, helps calm screaming and yelling types of tension, and with the entire B-complex helps improve the appetite, tone the muscles and help prevent nervous disorders.	watercress, brown rice, peaches, prunes, fresh string beans, soy beans, parseley, spinach, kale, rosehips and Jerusalem artichokes.
VITAMIN B_3	helps in excessive tiredness, falling hair, muscle cramps, muscle tone and as a general stimulant to the system.	parseley, potatoes and asparagus.
VITAMIN B_5	the entire B-complex helps to improve the appetite, tone the muscles, and acts as a general stimulant to the system.	grapefruit, oranges, strawberries, cauliflower and cabbage.

148

VITAMIN	USE	SOURCE
VITAMIN B_6	helps to prevent insomnia, oily skin, dizzyness, fatigue, stiffness of the joints, trembling of the limbs, protects against toxins in the system, and helps improve the appetite.	wheat germ, peas, carrots, spinach, egg yolks, potatoes, lemons, royal jelly, honey, broccoli, molasses, peanuts, rice, tuna, salmon, liver, sardines, soybeans and human milk.
VITAMIN B_8	the entire B-complex helps to stimulate the system, improve the appetite, tone the muscles, and help to prevent nervous disorders.	alfalfa and mint.
VITAMIN B_{12}	helps to regulate menstruation, improve the appetite, tone the muscles and help to prevent nervous disorders.	yeast cabbage, cauliflower, broccoli and honey.
BIOTIN	with the entire B-complex, helps to improve the appetite, tone the muscles, acts as a general stimulant to the system and helps to prevent nervous disorders.	lettuce, honey, cauliflower, spinach and grapefruit.
FOLIC ACID	aids digestion and the circulation of the blood.	parsley, potatoes, oranges, spinach and honey.
ISOTOL	with the entire B-complex, helps to improve the appetite, tone the muscles, acts as a general stimulant and helps to prevent nervous disorders.	kale, cauliflower, oranges, grapefruit and cauliflower.

VITAMIN	USE	SOURCE
NICOTINIC ACID	with the B-complex, helps to improve the appetite, tone the muscles, acts as a general stimulant and helps prevent nervous disorders.	wheat germ, fish, peas and garlic.
VITAMIN C	essential to healthy gums and teeth, acts to prevent scurvy and is also important to the nerves and for prevention of infections.	fresh oranges, grapefruit, lemons, tomatoes, cabbage, black currants, green peppers, nettles, cucumbers, rosehips, honey, violet leaves, yerba mate, Jerusalem artichokes, string beans, hibiscus, parseley, garlic, dandelion, black spruce, carrot, carrot leaves, prunes, raspberry leaves, lemons, spinach and all fruits.
VITAMIN D	necessary for proper growth of bones and production of good teeth and vision.	cod liver oils, fish liver oils, milk (very small amounts), honey, butter, cream, eggs and irradiated foods, lemon juice, spinach, apricots, wheat and sunshine.
VITAMIN E	strengthens reproductive faculties, muscle health, heart and circulatory disorders, oxygenates the body and lengthens cell life.	lettuce, parseley, pears, spinach, mustard leaves, potatoes, leeks, lemons, carrots, cucumbers, wheat germ, corn oil, turnips, turnip leaves, cottonseed oil, brown rice, nettles, nuts, legumes, honey, kale, raspberry leaves and pumpkin seeds.

VITAMIN	USE	SOURCE
VITAMIN F	required by the blood for co-agulation.	apples, apple pits, alfalfa, olive oil, orange peels, grapes, cherries, and all green vegetables.
VITAMIN G	regarded as an aid to general health with special importance for the skin. Also important in the coagulation of the blood and the stomach processes.	cheese, eggs, liver, brains, greens, cereal, potatoes, raspberry leaves, cranberries and alfalfa.
VITAMIN H	nourishes the glands and helps sulfur assimilate into the system.	mushrooms
VITAMIN K	essential in the clotting ability of the blood.	shepherd's purse, apple pits, parsley, brown rice, all greens, alfalfa, rosehips, cabbage, spinach, turnips and carrots.
VITAMIN P	important to the well-being of every cell in the body, helps coagulation of the blood, capillary action, helps in the control of hemorrhaging and to throw off body wastes.	rosehips, alfalfa, black berries, plums, white grapefruit, orange peels, lemons, grapes, black currants, apricots, carrots, spinach, rutin, cherries and apple pits.

HAND CHART

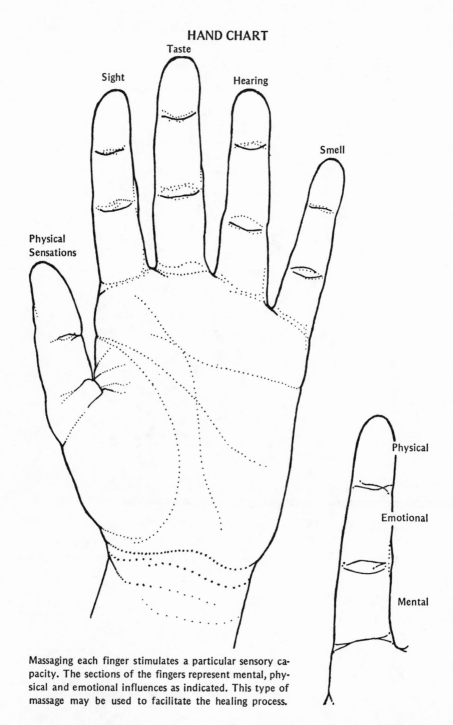

Massaging each finger stimulates a particular sensory capacity. The sections of the fingers represent mental, physical and emotional influences as indicated. This type of massage may be used to facilitate the healing process.

HERBAL SOURCES

If you are in the market for herbs which your local grocery or health food store doesn't have and you don't know enough to recognize the ones you need growing wild, there are several excellent herb stores located in different parts of the country. Here are some and what they have to offer:

Indiana Botanic Gardens
P.O. Box 5
Hammond, Indiana 46325

The Indiana Botanic Gardens grow and stock thousands of different herbs, seeds and some plants, but buying plants is tricky if you live across state lines. If you need an herb list, almanac, or just want information they will answer you promptly and send you what they have. If the herbs you need are not on their list write to them anyway, as they have found herbs for me which are listed in their catalogues under entirely different names. The Indiana Botanic Gardens grow most of their own herbs and the supply is fresh and fairly inexpensive.

Lhasa Karnak Herb Company
2513 Telegraph Avenue
Berkeley, California 94704

Lhasa Karnak stocks herbs, spices, ginseng and even herbal smoking mixtures and tea strainers. They sell both large and small quantities and will help you find what you need if they don't have it. Since I live near Lhasa Karnak, I use this supplier most often and have been quite happy with the freshness and quality of the herbs, expecially imported herbs, the quality of which can vary quite a bit. They have a complete catalogue of the products they stock which is available for $.25 and is revised and updated often. Buying from them in person, prices are low and the variety high.

World Wide Herbs, Ltd.
11 St. Catharines East
Montreal 129, Quebec

I have never used this source, but it has been recommended to me. This herb seller also buys herbs and sells tinctures, extracts and the like. Write for their catalogue at the above address.

A. Nelson & Company, Ltd.
Homeopathic Pharmacy
73 Duke Street
Grosvenor Square
London, W1M, 6BY
England

A. Nelson & Company stocks all the Bach remedies and some other herbal remedies and tinctures. They have a small package of information which lists their products and how to order for foreign shipment available upon request.

Culpeper Ltd.
21 Bruton Street
London W1 x 8DS
England

Culpeper Limited is run by the Society of Herbalists and carries herbal blends and cosmetics, as well as tonics and other herbal products. Their catalogue and prices are available from the above address.

Nature's Herbs
281 Ellis Street
San Francisco, California 94102

Nature's Herbs is a pharmacy which specializes in botanicals. They've been in business since 1915 and will mail order anywhere in the world. This outlet contains the largest variety on the West Coast and the people are knowledgeable and friendly. Write or call them for more information.

STAMPS Apothecary
33 Van Buren
Eureka Springs, Arkansas 72632

Owned by a registered pharmacist who specializes in over 300 herbs and oils as well as a complete line of homeopathic medicines, vitamins, etc. Mail order information is available from the above address.

If, when you write or visit these suppliers, you ask for seed lists you can start to grow your own herbs and guarantee their availability and freshness.

REFERENCES

REFERENCES

The books listed below are by no means the total of those available, but they are books I have used and like.

Edward Bach, **Heal Thyself**, C. W. Daniel, Company, Ltd., London, England

Edwin F. Bowers, Wm. H. Fitzgerald and George Starr White, **Zone Therapy**, I. W. Long, publisher, Columbus, Ohio

Philip M. Chancellor, editor, **Handbook of Bach Remedies**, W. C. Daniel, Company, Ltd., London, England

Nicholas Culpeper, **Culpeper's Complete Herbal**, W. Foulsham and Company, Ltd., New York

Mrs. M. Grieve, **A Modern Herbal**, 2 volumes, Dover Publications, Inc., New York

Eunice D. Ingham, **Stories the Feet Can Tell**, Rochester, New York

Jethro Kloss, **Back to Eden**, Lifeline Books, Santa Barbara, California

J. I. Rodale, **Encyclopedia of Common Diseases**, Rodale Books, Inc., Pennsylvania

Theosophical Research Center, **The Mystery of Healing**, Quest Books, Wheatton, Illinois

James Terrel, Marcia Terrel and Robert Wilborn, **Handbook of Iridiagnosis and Rational Therapy**, Health Research, Mokelumne Hill, California.

Aubrey T. Westlake, **The Pattern of Health**, Shambhala, Berkeley and London

INDEX

INDEX

A

Vitamin A- 32, 40, 44, 51, 52, 57, 65, 74, 75, 90, 93, 103, 105, 138, 139, 148.
abscesses- 117, 119.
acacia- 121.
acid- 16, 54, 71.
Acidosis- see Arthritis
acne- 104-106.
adder's tongue- 61..
adrenal glands- 16, 77, 79, 82.
adrenalin- 24, 128.
aging- 28, 79.
agrimony- 47, 85, 99.
alcohol- 16, 27, 32, 101.
alcoholism- 27, 32.
alder bark- 124.
ale- 123.
alfalfa- 16, 17, 44, 57, 62, 65, 67, 75, 76, 87, 88, 90, 102, 11, 119, 123, 128, 132.
alkaline- 16, 32.
allergies- 39, 54.
alloes- 108, 120.
allspice- 50.
almonds- 100.
almond oil- 67.
almond meal- 105.
alum- 69, 72, 91, 92, 115.
American Century- 32.
American cowslip- 38.
angelica- 28.
amino acids- 14.
animal diseases- 137-142.
animal fats- 89.
animal cancer- 139.
anise- 34, 48.
antibiotics and animals- 140.
ants- 90.
anus- 20, 56.
apple- 20, 40, 61, 62, 64, 78, 84, 89, 98.
apple cider vinegar- 59, 68, 112.
apple seeds- 20.
apricots- 23, 33, 39, 40, 43, 55, 105, 106.
arbutis- 96.
archangel- 44.

arnica- 109.
arsenic poisoning- 130, 131.
arteriolsclerosis- 86.
arteries- 83, 87,
arthritis- 16-19.
artichokes- 40, 52, 100, 101.
arrhythmic heartbeat- 77.
asafetida- 88.
ash- 54.
asparagus- 52, 93.
asparin- 80.
arsesmart. 121.
asthma- 39-44.
athlete's foot- 106-107.
attitude- 20, 122.
autism- 27.
avens herb- 37, 93, 106.
avocadoes- 57, 76.

B

vitamin B- 17, 31,32, 40, 41, 31, 32, 40, 41, 51, 54, 55, 64, 65, 66, 73, 76, 78, 91, 97, 100, 103, 105, 112, 124, 138-141,148, 149.
baby, eyewash- 63.
baby, teething- 121.
Bach, Edward- 128.
backaches- 8, 19, 20.
bacon fat- 20, 139.
bacteria- 119.
bags under the eyes- 62.
bakery products- 123.
baking soda- 80, 130, 131.
balm leaves- 18, 51, 98, 101.
bamboo shoots- 52, 54, 125.
bananas- 18, 101, 123.
barberry- 37.
barley- 23, 36, 42, 51, 55, 76, 89, 120, 124.
basil- 21, 73, 91.
basillion- 93.
basswood- 25, 80.
bay leaves- 49, 91, 112.
bayberry- 37.

bean juice- 17
bean sprouts- 52.
beans- 29, 47, 75, 78.
bearsfoot- 53.
bedwetting- 95.
beechdrops- 109.
bed sores- 107.
bee stings- 90.
beef broth- 126.
beer- 92, 95, 123.
beeswax- 18.
beets- 29, 32, 41, 44, 79, 84, 88, 89, 90, 93, 97, 98, 108, 141.
bell peppers- 84, 97.
berry juice- 34, 79.
bicarbonate of soda- 91.
bile- 97, 99.
bile, retention- 99.
bileberry- 47, 55.
bioflavoids- 33.
birch bark- 95.
birth- 75, 140
birth, after- 140.
birth control- 70.
birthwort- 18, 73.
biscuits- 123.
bistort- 37.
bites- 14, 141.
bitter root- 101.
bittersweet- 106.
black cohosh 33, 73,
black elder bark - 53.
black eye- 62, 63.
black hellborn- 73.
black spots before the eyes- 64.
black tea- 16, 36, 47.
blackberries- 107.
blackheads- 104, 105.
bladder, obstructions- 95.
bladder, stones- 93.
bladder, ulcers- 51.
bladderwrack-54.
bleeding-87, 97, 140,
bleeding of piles and hemorrhoids- 56
blemishes- 104.
blessed thistle- 18.

blindness- 63, 64.
blistering, cancer- 30, 66.
blood blisters- 106.
blood cells- 13, 18, 31, 59, 98, 99.
blood cleansers- 67.
blood clots- 84, 86, 130.
blood pressure- 80, 87, 88, 89.
blood root- 39, 50, 109, 110, 112.
blood shot eyes- 59, 64.
blue flag- 56, 71, 98, 105.
blueberries- 43, 55, 78.
blurred vision-65.
boils- 106, 107.
bones-97.
bone marrow- 31.
bones, broken- 13
bones, softening- 128.
bone meal-128.
bowels- 52, 54, 75, 76, 90, 105.
boxleaf- 99, 100.
brain-20-28.
brain cells-23.
brain, damage- 28.
brain tumors-31.
bran-76.
bread, unhulled- 103.
breaking a fast- 136.
breasts- 75, 117.
breasts, caked -75.
breasts, cancer- see Cancer.
breathing exercises for lung cancer-30.
brewer's yeast- 18, 79, 81, 105, 107, 110, 138, 139.
Bright's disease- 34.
broccoli- 52, 57, 75, 116.
bronchial asthma- 37.
bronchial congestion and bronchitis- 38, 40, 41, 42.
brown rice- 84, 89
brown sugar- 32, 84, 90.
bruises- 13, 104, 107.
bruises to the eyes- 62.
bryony- 42, 44, 45.
buchue- 94, 95.
buck bean- 50.
buckwheat- 82, 84.

bugle- 27, 78.
bugs, animal- 140.
bugs, plants- 141.
bullweed- 131.
bumps on the knuckles- 17, 119.
bunions- 108-109.
burns- 109.
burdock- 47, 85, 109, 117.
bursitis- 16.
butcher's broom- 94.

C
vitamin C- 18, 20, 22, 23, 26, 27, 28,
31, 32, 33, 39, 40, 51, 52, 53, 57, 59,
65, 74, 75, 81, 82, 84, 90, 91, 93, 94,
96, 97, 100, 105, 119, 124, 128, 129,
130 and appendices.
cabbage- 51, 75.
cabbage, skunk- 41.
caffeine-65.
caladine greater- 65.
calamint- 25, 118, 119.
calamus -46.
calcium- 16, 20, 21, 23, 26, 27, 35, 59,
62, 65, 68, 72, 73, 89, 102, 103, 104,
105, 115, 119 and appendices.
calluses- 16, 66, 108.
calories-122.
camomile- 22, 48, 89, 72, 91, 96, 103,
118, 121, 125, 140.
Canada thistle- 55.
cancer- 28-31, 104.
cancer, animal-139.
cancerillo- 109.
cankers- 37.
canned fruit- 39, 89.
capsicum- see cayenne.
caraway- 20, 34, 95, 96.
carbohydrates- 135.
carbuncles- 111.
cardamon seeds- 26, 49, 98.
carob- 22, 138.
carrot- 23, 26, 29, 30, 32, 40, 43, 44,
51, 52, 57, 64, 79, 87, 88, 89, 93, 97,
98, 105, 111, 131.
cascara bark- 53.

cashews- 52.
castor oil- 93, 108, 126.
cataracts- 65, see Eyes.
catnip- 27.
cats- 138.
cauliflower- 75;
cavities- 119.
cayenne- 18, 20, 21, 23, 27, 35, 59, 62, 65,
72, 73, 89, 102, 103, 104, 105, 115,
119.
cedar bark- 124.
celery- 23, 29, 40, 51, 52, 79, 87, 88,
98, 100, 102, 105, 131, 138.
cell salts- 39, 111.
cereal- 55, 123.
camphor-phenique- 64, 92, 106, 111.
chapped eyelids- 63.
chapped hands- 13, 105.
charcoal- 46, 109, 113.
cheese- 29, 71, 156,
chervil- 38.
chest infections- 40, 42, 45, 46, 131.
chemicals- 7, 101.
chemical medications- 12.
cholesterol- 69, 83, 96.
chlorine- see appendices.
chlorinated water- 134.
chronic sleeplessness- 21.
Chronic and Degenerative diseases- 31-
35.
cherry- 17, 39, 84, 97.
cherry bark- 124.
chewing- 7.
chia seeds- 21.
chicken- 64, 123, 126.
chickweed- 33, 44, 46, 79, 124.
chipweed- 20.
chiropractor- 19, 131.
chives- 19, 89.
cider vinegar- 18.
cigarettes- ashes- 139.
cinnamon- 47.
cinquefoil- 75.
circles under the eyes- 62.
circulation-59, 71, 80, 81-86, 128.
cirrhosis-101, 102.

citronella 67, 92.
citrus juice- 57, 99.
clammy skin- 116.
clay- 109.
cleansers, eye- 63, see Eye.
cleansers, glands- see Glands.
cleansers, liver- see Liver and Spleen.
Cleaver's herb-49, 94, 96, 106, 112, 123.
clover- 6, 37, 49, 67, 124.
cloves- 22, 52, 120.
colon- 54, see Digestive System.
cane sugar- 7.
cocoabutter - 33.
coconuts- 29, 98, 116.
cod liver oil- 17.
coffee- 2, 16, 32, 65, 98, 142.
congestion- 35-37, 80, 97, 139.
cohosh, black- 33.
cold all the time- 77, feet and hands-89, 67, 115, 117.
colds- 6, 35-46.
cold sores- 111.
colic- 47, 48.
colitis- 52, 54.
coltsfoot- 39, 42.
colombo- 49.
comdurango- 51.
comfrey- 13, 16, 37, 42, 52, 54, 30, 31, 43, 75, 76, 81, 94, 102, 104,105, 108, 109. 115, 118, 129, 138, 140, 141.
confusion- see Brain.
conception- 75.
conjunctivitis- 62, animal-139.
constipation- 52-54.
contractions- 75.
contraception- 69, 70.
convulsions- 24.
complexion- 105, cleansers-105.
copper- 105 and appendices.
coriander- 48.
corn oil- 138.
corn meal- 84, 89, 115.
corn silk- 17, 61, 94, 95.
corns- 16, 66, 108.
corneal ulcers- 65.
cortex, brain- 23, 28.

cortisone, natural- 16, chemical-128.
cottage cheese- 71, 135, 138, 140.
contagious diseases- 132.
cottonroot- 73.
cottonseed oil- 18.
coughs- 35-46.
counseling- 20.
crackers- 123.
cramps- 49, 50, 68, 72, 73, 74, 132.
cranberries- 22, 30, 31.
cream- 49, 63, 109.
cucumbers- 22, 29, 32, 43, 44, 51, 52, 53, 62, 74, 78, 80, 83, 93, 98, 100, 102, 103, 106, 112.
cudweed- 36.
currants, red and black- 34, 107.
cuticles- 115.
cut worms- 142.
cysts- 31, 64, 75.

D

vitamin D- 16, 21, 27, 35, 59, 70, 75, 102, 109.
dandelion- 19, 38, 43, 54, 63, 71, 85, 90, 93, 94, 96, 98, 99, 100, 110, 112.
dandruff- 112.
darnel- 35.
dates- 84.
deafness- 57, 58, 59.
decay, tooth- 29, 112.
decongestant- 35.
degenerative diseases 32-35.
dehydration, in animals- 138.
delirium tremens (DT's)- 27.
depression- 26, 122, in animals- 138.
devil's walking stick- 58.
devitalized foods- 7.
diabetes- 100, 101.
diaper rash- 110.
diarrhea- 55, animal-138.
diet- 29, 86, 87, 88, 122, for colds-35.
digestion- 46-57, 50, 66, 76, 119, 135, animal-138-139.
dill- 20, 49, 132.
dimming of sight- 63.
discharge, vaginal-65, 66.

dissatisfaction- 6.
dock, yellow- 67, 85, 113, 120, 131.
dodder- 100, 26.
dogwood, swamp- 55.
dolomite- 24, 31, 72, 81, 102, 128.
dong kwei- 72.
douche- 72.
dragon flowers- 63.
drinking with meals- 8, 49.
dropsy- 34.
dry skin- 113, 116, 117.
dulse- 22, 67, 77, 119.
dysentery- 55.
dyspepsia- 55.

E
vitamin E-26, 28, 31, 40, 51, 52, 60,
75, 76, 81, 82, 84, 86, 88, 89, 93, 94,
102, 105, 106, 118, 139, 140 and appendices.
earaches- 58.
ear mites- 92.
ears- 57-59.
eating- 7.
eczema- 112, 113, pets- 139.
edema- 34.
eggs- 23, 29, 40, 64, 103, 108, 110,
112, 115, 118.
elderberry- 37, 67, 107.
elder bark- 53, 55, 56.
elderly- 49, 55.
elimination- 54.
elm bark- 46, 131.
emergency procedures- 128-132.
emotional disturbance-20-28.
emphysema 42, 44, 45.
endive- 100.
endrocrine glands- 72, 77, 103.
enemas- 83.
energy foods- 52, 77, 89.
enzymes- 47, 49.
epilepsy-24, 34.
epsom salts- 35.
equilibrium- 45.
eruptions- see Skin.
estrogen- 72.

eyes-59-65, bags under-62, black eyes-
63, bloodshot- 64, bruised- 64, blurring-
63, cataracts- 64, 65, chapped-63, cysts-
64, glaucoma- 64, 65, infection- 62,
night blindness- 64, red eyes- 63, to
strengthen- 60, 61, 62, stys- 64, sun-
burned- 64.
eucalyptus- 44, 91, 92, 140, 141.
evaporated milk- 62.
exercise- 9, 122.
exhaustion- 40.
expectorants- see Colds and Coughs.
expel worms- 125.
external cancer- 28- 30.

F
vitamin F- 31, 64, and appendices.
fainting- 33.
fallen arches- 68.
falling sickness- 34.
far-sightedness- 59.
fasting- 134-136, how to break a fast-
135, 136, and each chapter for specific fasts.
fat deposits- 83, storage- see Liver section.
fatigue- 23, 45.
fatty acids- 31.
fear- 6.
feet and legs- 20, 66-69, 77, 87, 106,
107, 117.
female- 69-77, animal pregnancy- 139.
fennel- 33, 34, 48, 71, 72, 73, 74, 75,
76, 90, 95, 116, 124, 131.
fenugreek- 42, 43.
fern, root- 126, sword fern- 114.
fetus- 76.
fever- 37, 38.
feverweed- 45.
fibrillation- see Heart and Circulation.
figs- 54, 78, 84, 113, 118, 120.
fingers- 114, 115.
fish- 25, 44, 64.
fit root-26, 61, 83.
flatulance- 48.
flaxseed- 41, 52, 54, 62, 79, 94, 131, 141.

fleas- 91, 92, flea collars- 140.
flour, white- 7, 103.
flowers- 141, flower pumice- 119.
flu- 6, 39, 42.
food, devitalized- 7.
food, poisoning- 130.
forgetfulness- 23.
frequent urination- 95, 96.
frost bite- 69, 105.
fruit- combinations of 7, 8, 106, 107.
fruit, canned- 123.
fungus- see athlete's foot.

G

vitamin G- 32, 52, 74, 75.
gallstones- 96.
gangrene- 113.
gargle- 36, 37, 46, 47, 120.
garlic- 13, 21, 31, 36, 40, 41, 42, 43,
50, 55, 75, 82, 83, 86, 88, 94, 107,
113, 114, 115, 125, animals-139-141.
gas- 7,8, causes; 46, 47, 48, 49, 53, 75,
80, animal gas-139.
gastritis- 49.
gelatin- 83, 123.
genitals-118, see Male.
gentian- 49, 51, 98.
giant Solomon seal root- 71.
ginger- 33, 38, 48, 55, 60, 77, 80.
ginseng 41, 72, 104.
glands- system 77-79, 22, and skin 103,
male glands- 102.
glandular swelling- 38, 42.
glaucoma- 65.
gluten foods- 81, 83, 122.
goat milk- 32, 35, 62, 123, for pets-139.
golden seal- 65, 80, 99, 109, 110, 112,
114, 121.
gout- 18, 19, 69.
goutweed- 19.
grains- 91, 141.
grape brandy- 42.
grapefruit- 59, 85, for fever- 45.
grape leaves, Oregon- 109.
grapevine juice- 63, grapes- 30, 31, 78, 89,
gravels- 96.

Grave's disease- 32.
green beans- 52.
green elder- 51.
green peppers- 33,
green soap- 68, 93, 107.
grendelia- 113.
grey hair- 115.
ground ivy- 17, 26, 80.
growth- 77, skin growths 108, 109,
animal growths- 139.
gulping foods and liquids- 117, see Gas
gum camphor- 18.
gum plant- 113.
gum styrax- 93.
gums and teeth- 119-121.

H

hair, falling out- 140.
hallucinations- 27.
halitosis- 46.
hardboiled eggs- 112.
hare lettuce- 104.
hate- 6.
hawthorne- 26, 98.
haychaff and arthritis- 17.
hayfever- 39.
head- 131.
headaches- 7, 43, 80-81, 89.
heart- 21, 81-86.
heart attacks- 83.
heart beat- 83.
heart muscle disease- 84.
heart palpitations- 89.
heart strain- 122.
heartburn- 48, 50, also see Gas.
hemorrhaging- 28, 130.
hemorrhoids- 57.
hepatitis- 99, 100.
hesperidin (vitamin P) 18, 33, 34, 108,
130 and appendices.
herbal remedies, uses of- 12.
herbs- 20, 141.
hernias- 13.
herpes - 111.
hiccups- 49, 132.

high blood pressure- 81, 87-90, also see Heart and Circulatory System section.
hives- 113.
holly seeds- 25.
honey- 13, 18, 27, 29, 35, 36, 38, 41, 44, 45, 46, 48, 73, 74, 78, 79, 80, 89, 90, 95, 116, 120, 131.
honeysuckle- 35, 40, 58, 90, 117.
hops- 23.
horehound- 43, 44, 49, 58, 117.
hormones- 70, 86, 97, 102, 123.
horsebain- 47.
horse meat, and animals- 138.
horseradish- 38, 44, 49, 95.
horsetail herb- 20, 29, 61.
hot flashes- 54.
hysterectomy- 69, 72.
huckleberry- 101.
human milk- 52.
hydrogen- see appendices.
hydrogen-peroxide- 58.
hypoglycemia- 89, 90.
hyssop- 42, 47, 58, 117.
hysteria- 26, also see Brain section.

I
ice cream- 123.
impotency- 104.
increase flow of urine- 94, 95.
indigestion- 8, 49, 50.
infants- 55.
infections- 13, 57, 58, 60, 61, 62, 63, also, see ailment by name.
infertility- 74.
inflammation- 16, prostate-103.
influenza- 45.
ingrown nails- 69, 115.
insanity- 25.
insects- 90-93, bites- see skin, on pets- 141.
insomnia- 21, 22.
insulin- 100, see diabetes.
internal cancer- 29-31.
internal worms- 125.
intestinal disorders- see digestion.
intestinal tract- 104, 135.

iron- 23, 27, 102, 103, 105, and appendices.
irritation- kidney- 94.
Irish moss- 77.
Irisdiagnosis- 59.
itch, from kidney irritations- 93, from liver conditions- 99, from skin rashes, bites- 113, pets- 137-142, vaginal-70.
ivy, poison-104, 114.
ivy, ground- 17, 20, 26, 38, 43, 50, 62, 80, 82, 100.

J
jaborandi- 42.
jam- 123.
jasmine- 29, 35.
jaundice- 99, 100, animal-140.
Jerusalem artichokes- 40, 52, 100, 101.
jewel weed- 114.
joint pain, arthritis- 16, 17.
juices, fresh vegetable- 29, 30, 31, for fasting- 134-136, for the skin- 105, for weight loss- 123, also see ailment and recommended diet.
juices, continued. weight loss- 123, also see ailment for recommended diet.
juice, plant- for insect repellent-135.
juniper berries- 21, 34, 56, 93, 94, 95, 102, 135, 142.

K
vitamin K- 32, 52, 74, 93, and appendices.
kelp- 23, 47, 53, 111, and pets- 138.
kidney- 8, 12, 42, 64, 82, 93, 95, 104, 93-97, and low back pain- 19.
kidney stone- 93, 96.
knee, out of place- 128.
knotgrass- 76, 114.
knuckles, bumps on- 17.
knuckles, popping- 87.

L
labor- 75.
lanolin- 44, 92, 105.
lard- 18, 19, 63, 107, 113.

larkspur- 92.
lavender flowers- 18, 33.
laxatives- 52, see Digestion.
laryngitis- 36, 47.
lead colic- 50.
lecithin- 16, 20, 33, 69, 76, 83, 86, 92, 96, 122.
leeks- 118.
leg cramps- 68.
lemon juice- 21, 22, 23, 34, 36, 42, 44, 47, 49, 54, 61, 64, 68, 78, 81, 86, 98, 99, 101, 105, 108, 113, 116, 124, 13, 14.
lemon rind- 119.
lentils- 29, 78.
leprosy- 118, 119.
lettuce- 23, 52, 123.
lettuce juice- 100, 102.
leukemia- 31.
leucorrhia - 72.
lice- 92.
licorice- 39, 41, 52, 72, 74.
linden flowers- 67.
life everlasting herb- 41.
limes-97, 118, and appendices.
lime juice- 119.
liniment- 18, 113, 114.
liver- 8, 12, 30, 39, 42, 82, 97-102.
liver, pets- 140.
lobelia- 106.
lockjaw- 68, pet lockjaw- 141.
loss of weight- 122, 123, 124.
lotion, skin- 105.
lovage- 48, 50.
low blood pressure- 87-90.
low energy- 77.
lucerne herb- 17.
lumbar- 19.
lungs- 30, colds- 40, 41, 42, 46, also see Cancer.
lungwort- 23, 38.

M

magnesium- 16, 24, 27, 29, 35, 39, 41, 72, 74, 89, 102, 104, 105, 115.

maidenhair- 60.
malaria- 42.
males- 102-104.
malt- 118.
malt vinegar- 71, 120.
mammary glands- 76.
mandrake- 82.
manic depression- 27.
mange- 139.
mangoes- 52, 93.
manzanita- 92.
marigold- 20, 107.
marrow, bone- 89.
marshmallow- 96.
massage- 20, 66, 68, 70, 94, 102, 120.
masterwort- 28, 40, 53.
may apples- 54, 85, 100.
may flowers- 26, 42.
mayonaise- 115.
meadowsweet- 49.
measles- 6.
meat and cancer- 29.
meat tenderizer- 91.
melancoly- 26.
mellilot -43, 103.
meningitis-35. ·
menopause- 74.
menstruation, decrease flow- 73.
menstruation- induce suppressed-73, 74.
mental attitude- 28, 122, and cancer- see Cancer.
mental retardation- 28.
mezereum -18.
metabolism- 122, 123, also see Glandular System.
milk-8, 35, 39, 55, 107, 118, evaporated- 62, sour- 134.
milkweed- 95, 118.
millet- 89.
minerals- 7, 13, 28, and appendices.
mind- 19.
mint- 91, 112, 140.
miscarriage- 74, 75.
mites, ear- 58, pests- 91.
mongolism- 28.
monkshood- 38, 108, 115.

mononeucleosis- 40.
morning sickness- 76.
mosquitoes- 92.
moths- 91, on plants-141.
mouse ear herb- 95, 96.
mouseroot- 36.
mouth- 46, paralysis-33, ulcers-36.
mucous- 35, 37, 39, 41, 42, 43, 52, 118,
also see Colds and Coughs.
mucous membranes- 63, 78.
mud- 90.
mugwort- 23, 73.
mullien 42, 56, 58, 59, 69, 120.
multiple sclerosis- 31.
mumps- 6.
muscle cramps- 68, 132.
mucles spasms- 31.
muscle stiffness- 114.
muscle strength- 27.
muscle meats- 89.
muscular dystrophy- 31, 32.
mushrooms- 78, see vitamin H.
mustard 16, 18, 124, greens-82, seeds-
49.
mycelin- 31.
myrrh -26, 121.

N
nails- 114, 115.
nasal congestion - 44, cavity- 44, 110.
naturopath- 19, see Authors.
nausea- 53, 76, 99.
neck collars- 131.
neck vertebrae- 131.
negativity- 131, see Cancer.
nerve root- 22.
nervousness- 26, 27, 67, and high
blood pressure- 88, 89.
nerves- 21, 66-69.
nettles- 16, 42, 85, 88, 104, 114, 131.
neuritis- 18, see Arthritis.
niacin- 102, see appendices.
nicotinic poisoning-43.
nicotinic acid- 90, appendices.
night blindness- 64, 112.
noises in the ears- 57.

non-glue foods- 122.
nosebleeds- 87.
nostrils, to check for worms- 125.
nursing mothers- 76, also see Pets and
Plants.
nutmeg- 22, 93.
nuts- 78, 83, 97, 103.

O
oak bark- 72.
oat flour- 89.
oat groats- 23, 82, 111.
oats- 79, 87.
oatstraw- 17, 29, 67,   , 79, 86, 94, 104.
obstruction in digestive tract- 53, in
other organs, see specific organ.
odor, breath- 46
odor, from cancer decay- 29.
okra- 83, 106.
ointment- 59.
oily skin- 105, 116, 117.
old sores- 107.
olive oil- 54, 58, 59, 96, 99, 101, 116,
121, 125.
onions- 21, 41, 43, 48, 58, 59, 75, 79,
91, 93.
open sores- 105.
open wounds- 108.
orache- 114.
oranges- 8, 18, 21, 45, 64, 65, 81, 134,
orange peels- 49, 91.
organ meat- 89.
osteopath- 19, 131.
ovaries- 70, see Female section.
over eating- 7, 55, 56, 125.
overweight- 122.
oxygen- 26, 86, 106, 112, also see appendices.

P
vitamin P- 18, 32, 33, 63, 108, 130.
pain-see each organ. in ear- 57, 58, head-
80, 81, joints- 17, 18, lungs- 41.
palsy - 32.
pancreas- 31, 39, 81, 101, 128.
pansy   113.

pantothenic acid- 27, 52, 89, 107, 115.
also, see appendices.
papain- 125.
papaya- 47, 51, 54, 57, 61, 62, 125,
134.
paralysis- 28.
parasites- 92, 104.
parathyroid- 77, see Glandular System.
parkinson root- 113.
parseley- 17, 29, 40, 43, 44, 46, 48,
50, 51, 57, 59, 72, 81, 85, 87, 88, 97,
100, 119, 120, 131.
parsnips- 38, 97, 101.
passion flower- 26, 74, 88.
pasta- 123.
pastries- 81.
peanuts- 52, butter- 83.
peaches- 39, 84, 85, 87, 110.
pears- 84, 96.
peas- 90, 103, 138.
pecans- 16.
pelvis- 19.
pennyroyal- 37, 41, 73, 77, 91, for pets-
141.
peppergrass- 124.
peppermint- 18, 26, 27, 37, 49, 67, 72,
75, 110.
peppers, bell- 16, 32, 52, 82, 87, 97,
104, 105.
pepsin- 52.
peristalsis- 54, see Digestion.
peroxide- 14.
persimmons- 52, 54.
perspiration- 41.
pessimism- 26.
phlegm- 18, 42.
plebitis- 84, 85, 86.
phosphorus- 25, 74, 75, 85, 106, also
see appendices.
pigment- 62, 99, 100, 115.
pilewort- 56.
piles and hemorrhoids- 55, 56.
pineal gland- 79, see Glandular System.
pineapple- 118, 134.
pink eye- 62.
pimples- 104, 105, 106.

pit root- 72.
pituitary gland- 77, 79, 123, see also
Glandular System.
plague- 119.
plaintain- 19, 93.
plants- 141-142.
plum bark- 41.
plums- 33.
pleurisy-39, pleurisy root-82.
pneumonia- 42, 45.
pokeroot- 85.
polio- 33, 34.
pollen- 47.
pomegranates- 125.
popping joints- 17, 18, 128.
poppy seeds- 63, 109.
pork- 89.
poison ivy, oak- 104, 114.
poisoning- arsenic- 130, 131, food- 54,
radiation poisoning- 131.
potassium- 28, and appendices.
potatoes- 16, 61, 62, 67, chips- 123,
sweet- 123.
potency- 104.
poultice, how to prepare- 13.
poultry- 25, 83, 89.
pregnancy- 56, 75, 76, 115, animal-140.
pressure- in the head,- 80.
prickly ash- 33, 40, 50, 89, 117, 120.
primrose- 18, 33.
processed foods- 16, 77,.
progesterone- 72.
prolonged menstruation- 73.
protein- 48, 78, 103, see Cancer.
prostate, enlarged- 102, painful- 103.
proud flesh- 109.
prunes- 52, 134.
psoriasis- 115, also see eczema.
psychomatic illnesses- 6.
pumpkin seeds- 40, 53, 93, 102, 103,
126.
pursalane- 61.

Q
queen of the meadow root- 34.
queen's delight- 36, 84, 106.

quince seeds- 62, 111.

R

radiation poisoning- 131.
radishes-79, 93.
rapid heart- 83.
rashes- 13, 14, 109.
raspberry leaves- 37, 55, 68, 74, 75, 88, 90, 97, 110, 132, 140.
rectum- 46.
red blood cells- 16, see Liver and Spleen.
red clover- 30, 85, 105.
red eyes- 63.
red poppy- 90.
red sage- 26, 71, 98, 120.
relaxation- 22.
resistance- to disease, - 6.
respiration- 40, 44, see Coughs and Colds.
restlessness- 21, 26.
rhatany- 55, 112.
rhubarb- 79, 85.
rheumatism- 16, 17, 18.
rheumatoid arthritis- 18.
riboflavin- 65, 107, and appendices.
rice- 44, 105, 123, flour- 89, 123, and fish fast- 135.
ring-a-round - 114, 115.
ring worms- 125.
rocky mountain grape root- 96.
rolled oats- for pet pregnancies- 140.
rose bushes and bugs- 141.
rosehips- 22, 47, 65, 67.
rose oil- 57.
rosemary- 16, 18, 23, 60, 63, 73, 82, 91, rosemary oil for pets- 140.
rough skin- 13, 14, 116.
rue- 27, 35, 91, 131, oil- 92.
running sores- 117.
ruptures- 13.
rushes- 38, 74.
rutin- 59, 61, 65, 82, 84.
rye flour- 89.

S

sacred bark- 85.

saffron- 26, 83, 85, 93.
sage- 16, 23, 27, 33, 36, 47, 60, 90.
sagging breasts- 75, 117.
salads- 16, 99, 101.
saliva- 7, 77, 93, 113.
salivary glands- 7, 46.
salt- 16, 22, 63, 67, 77, 84, 87, 107, 135, 141.
sandalwood- 92.
sarcoidoses, see Cancer 30.
sarsaparilla- 19, 72, 74, 85, 115.
sassafras- 85, 89, 91, 105, 112, 113, 142.
sauerkraut- 99.
savory, summer- 57, 58.
saw palmetto- 76, 78.
scabies 93.
scalp- 112.
scaly skin- 117.
schizophrenia- 27.
sciatica-35.
scorpion- bites, stings- 131.
scrotum, bruised or swollen- 104.
seafood- 123.
seaweed- 81, 111, 119, 124.
sedatives- 28.
seizure-24, also see epilepsy.
senility- 28.
sesame oil- 64, 67, 76, 79, 107, 124.
sesame seeds- 78.
selenium- 86, 104 and appendices.
sex glands- 102-104, see Male and Female, and Glandular System.
sex hormones- 97.
shepherd's purse- 74, 124, 130.
sherbet-83.
shingles- 111.
shock- 128, to the stomach- 8.
shortness of breath- 38, also see emphysema.
sicklewort- 51, 57.
senna- 53, 54.
silicon- 86, 104, 107.
sinusitis-43,44.
skim milk- 83, 89.
skin- 104-119.

skin burns- 140, 141.
skin cancer- 109.
skin, rashes- 14, rough- 14.
skullcap- 21, 22, 49.
sleep- 21, see Brain section.
slippery elm bark- 46, 55, 85, 86, 131.
sluggishness- 8, and constipation- 77,
and fasting- 135, see also Glandular Section.
smoking- 32.
smoke inhalation- 131.
snake bite- 93, 131.
snakeroot- 25, 33, 50.
soak, for feet- 68.
soap, green- 68, non-alkaline- 105.
soapwort- 106.
sodium perborate- 46.
soft drinks- 123.
Solomon seal root- 45, 71, 108.
sore feet- 68, throats- 47.
sores- 75, 105, 106, 107, 111, 116, also
see individual ailment.
sour cream- 111.
sour dough bread- 30, 32.
soy beans- 20, 89, 100.
soy milk- 35, 36, 47, 78, 79, 123.
soy products (lecithin) - 93.
spanish onions- 43.
spasms- 26, 33, muscle- 130, see also
palsy and epilepsy.
spearmint- 110.
speedwell- 32, 41.
spices- 51.
spicewood- 84.
spiders- 135, see Insects.
spinach- 32, 40, 44, 52, 87, 93, 98, 99,
111, 131.
spinal column- 23, 28, also see Chronic
and Degenerative Diseases.
spirits of camphor- 62.
spittle- 109. 113.
spleen- 12, 26, 31, 39, 97-102, 135,
spleen and headaches- 80.
spots on the eyes- 64, on face and hands-
see Liver section, on the skin- 115.
sprains- 13, 132.

sprouts- 16.
squash- 87.
squawvine- 73, 75, 95.
starches- 7, 46, 89, 100.
sterility- 104.
stitches, to avoid- 109
stiffness of the joints- 16, 17, 18.
stinger, insect, scorpion, etc.- 90, 91, 113.
St. John's wort- 17, 37, 50, 71, 95.
stomach · 7, 8, 16, 46, 50, 80, aches-
7, lining- 51, tension- 20, 72, ulcers- 51.
strawberry- 47, 55, 99, and teeth-119.
strengthen eyes- 60, 61.
stress- 6, 51, 73, 87.
stretch marks- 76, 115.
string beans- 17, 100, 101.
strokes- see Heart section.
St. Vitus dance- 33.
stys- 118.
sugar- 7, 13, 16, 32, 39, 78, 83, 84, 87,
89, 100, 112, 115, 123.
sugar storage- see Liver and Spleen section.
sulfur- 111, 130, 131, and appendices.
sulfur flowers- 93.
sunburn- 109, sunburned eyes- 64.
sundew- 36, 118.
sunflower oil and seeds- 59, 64, 89, 117.
swamp dogwood- 55.
sweaty skin- 116.
sweet gum- 108.
sweet wine- 123.
swelling- 13, 98, in feet- 68, 118.
swollen eyes- 61.

T
tannic acid- 36, 46.
tansy-- 73, 125.
tapeworms- 125, 126.
tar- 139.
tartar, cream of- 113, 131.
tartar on the teeth- 119.
tea, black - 16.
tear gas- 131.
teething, baby- 121.
tension- 6, 9, 13, 20, 21, 22, 51, 61,

62, 80, 110, relieving- 66.
tetanus- 68, also see Pets.
thistle- 18, 55.
throat- 46, 131, sore- 35, 36, 37.
thrush- 36, 36,46, 121.
thuja- 18.
thyme- 47, 55, 91.
thyroid- 22, 77-79, 83, 119, and weight-
122.
ticks- 140.
tight shoes- 66, also see corns and calluses.
tighten the skin- 110.
tired eyes- 63.
toast, french- 123.
tobacco- 16, 68, 87, 92, 93, 101.
tobacco water and plants- 142.
toe stiffness-see gout.
toe nails, ingrown- 53-54.
tongue- 89, paralysis-33.
tonics- 23, see Glandular System and
Chronic Diseases.
tonsilitis- 42.
tomato juice- 8, 16, 99.
tomatoes- 16, 51, 54, 81.
toothaches and teeth- 13, 119, 120, 121.
toxemia- 24.
toxicity and backaches- 8, 19, 110, also
see kidney and bladder sections.
trembling limbs- 28, 33.
trench mouth- 121.
trick knees- 128.
tuberculosis- 40, 43, 44, 46.
tumors- 28-31.
turkey- 123.
turnips- 16, 82, 110.
turpentine- 18, 113.

U

ulcerative colitis- 52.
ulcers- eye- 65, mouth- 36, 46, 119, 120,
121, stomach- 50, 51.
ulcers, external- see skin.
unsaturated fats- 103.
upset stomach- 50.
urination- 94, 95, 96, 118,

urination, disorders of the prostate-102,
too frequent- 96.
urine, pregnant mare- 70.
uterus- 69, 70, 71, 72, 73, 77.

V

vagina- 72, see Female.
vaginal infections- 70, discharge-71, 72,
itches- 71.
valerian root- 18, 21, 50, 79.
varicose veins- 81, 86, see also Chronic
Diseases.
vaseline- 109, 116.
vegetables-13, 16, 20, 27, 80, 81, 82,
83, 86, 89, 104, 122, 123, 131, creamed-
123, raw for fasting- 134-141, oil-83.
vegetarians and   ginseng-104.
veins- 81, 87, see Heart and Circulatory
System.
vertebrae- 19.
vertigo- 95.
vervain- 25, 41, 54, 95.
vinegar- 17, 91, 106, 112, 113, malt-71.
violet leaves- 30, 44, 45, 61, 85, 105,
113.
vision- 59, see Eyes.
vitamins- 7, 13, see appendices for
uses and sources.

W

waffles- 81, 123.
walking- 122.
wall flowers- 100, 114.
walnut hulls- 28, 106, 125.
warts- 108. 118.
wash, for the eyes- 60.
wasp- 90. also see Insects.
water- 8, and backaches- 19-20, reten-
tion- see swollen eyes.
water brash- 46.
water cress- 29, 46, 103, 105, 107, 118.
water dock- 120.
watermelon- 78.
wax, in the ear- 59.
weight- 122-124, gain- 94, loss- 115;
wheat bran- 54, 79.

wheat germ- 16, 59, 78, 81, 103, 110. 113. 118.

wheat flour- 89, 113.
whiplash- 13, 131.
white ash- 34.
white flour- 7, 16, 32, 78.
white grapes- 17.
white flecks before the eyes-see Eyes. and Liver sections.
wild plum bark- 41.
will power- 122.
willow bark- 63, 69.
wine- 8, 123.
wintergreen- 18.
winter savory- 91.
wisdom teeth- 120.
witch hazel- 59, 61, 63, 107, 111, 120.
wood betony - 27.
worms- 125-126, in pets- 138.
worms, cut- 141-142.
wormseed- 73.
wormwood- 51, 54, 68, 92, 98, 125.
worry- 6.
wrinkles- 110.

X

Y
yams- 97, 100, 123.
yarrow- 34, 37, 58, 101, 104.
yeast- 16, 54, 138.
yeast infections- 71.
yerba mate- 41, 79, 124, 135.
yogurt- 71, 72, 111, 138, 140, goat yogurt- 62, 139, 140.

Z
zinc- 24, also see Feet and Epilepsy.
zinc sulfate- 93.
zucchini squash- 87.

ABOUT THE AUTHORS

Mildred Jackson, N.D. (naturopathic doctor) and Terri Teague, N.D. (G.B.) live in the San Francisco Bay Area. They have co-authored a second book entitled **Mental Birth Control.**

Mildred Jackson is a naturopathic doctor practicing in Albany, California. Her varied experiences include work in obesity clinics, convalescent hospitals, with undernourished children, and more than 25 years of private practice. Mildred has studied both drugless and chemical nursing, has taken three years of dental schooling and more than 300 courses in various types of healing, including iridiagnosis, color and flower healing, American, European, and Eastern herbalism and massage. In addition to her private practice, Mildred teaches a weekly class in alternative healing.

In addition to earning a naturopathy doctorate from Great Britain, Terri K. Teague has also received her doctorate in chiropractic from Life Chiropractic College-West, San Lorenzo, California. She has counseled emotionally disturbed adults, taught classes in alternative healing methods at several Bay Area institutions, and has been a featured guest author on radio and television talk shows. Her undergraduate studies were completed at Lenoir Rhyne College in Hickory, North Carolina, where she received her BA.

Mildred and Terri have most recently given lectures for the Wholistic Health and Nutrition Institute of Mill Valley, CA, the Berkeley Holistic Health Center and retreats sponsored by the California School of Herbal Studies in Guerneville. Articles have been published in various magazines such as *Alternatives, Well Being,* and *Rain: Journal of Appropriate Technology.*

NOTES

Gift Certificate

This copy of

is sent to you by

Lawton-Teague Publications
P.O. Box 12353
Oakland, CA 94604

Gift Certificate

This copy of

is sent to you by

Lawton-Teague Publications
P.O. Box 12353
Oakland, CA 94604

ORDER FORM

LAWTON-TEAGUE PUBLICATIONS
P. O. Box 12353
Oakland, CA 94604

THE HANDBOOK OF ALTERNATIVES TO CHEMICAL MEDICINE
by Mildred Jackson, N.D. and Terri Teague, N.D. (G.B.)

176pp, 5¼x8½, perfectbound, **$6.95**

THE HANDBOOK is a guide to maintaining health through herbal and other types of alternative methods for whatever ails you. Included are chapters on emergency procedures, fasting, plants, and pets, and numerous diagrams and appendices.

MENTAL BIRTH CONTROL
by Mildred Jackson, N.D. and Terri Teague, N.D. (G.B.)

64pp, 5½x8½, perfectbound, **$3.00**

Our new book for men/women/or couples who wish to make conception a conscious decision. MENTAL BIRTH CONTROL explains what mental birth control is, how it works, and gives some suggestions about how to practice it. Also included are personal experiences of six persons currently practicing mental birth control within various lifestyles and relationships. MENTAL BIRTH CONTROL contains information on how to conceive as well as how to prevent conception.

	QUANTITY	TOTAL
The Handbook of Alternatives to Chemical Medicine .... @ $6.95		
Mental Birth Control .... @ $3.00		
Tax (California Residents Only)		
Shipping ($1.00 Minimum 1 book + 50¢ each additional book .... to same address		
TOTAL ENCLOSED ..		

Check if Gift ☐ — Send To·

Name _____

Address (Street) _____

City, State, Zip _____

Ship To: (please print)

Name _____

Address (Street) _____

City, State, Zip _____

Allow 4 - 6 weeks for delivery.   Make checks to: Teague/Jackson.   —   Please pay in U.S. currency only.